Atlas of Gynaecological Diagnosis

Atlas of Gynaecological Diagnosis

Abdel Fattah Youssef

Professor and Ex-Chairman, Department of Obstetrics
and Gynaecology, Cairo University
Senior Gynaecological Surgeon, Kasr El Aini Hospital,
Cairo, Egypt

CHURCHILL LIVINGSTONE
EDINBURGH LONDON MELBOURNE AND NEW YORK 1984

CHURCHILL LIVINGSTONE
Medical Division of Longman Group Limited

Distributed in the United States of America by Churchill
Livingstone Inc., 1560 Broadway, New York, N.Y. 10036, and
by associated companies, branches and representatives
throughout the world.

First published 1984

ISBN 0 443 03018 9

British Library Cataloguing in Publication Data

Youssef, Abdel Fattah.
    Atlas of gynaecological diagnosis.
    1. Gynecology
    I. Title
    618.1   RG101

Library of Congress Cataloging in Publication Data

Youssef, Abdel Fattah.
    Atlas of gynaecological diagnosis.

    1. Women—Diseases—Diagnosis—Atlases. I. Title.
[DNLM: 1. Genital diseases, Female—Diagnosis—Atlases.
WP 17 Y83a]
RG107.Y68   1983   618.1'075   83-14437

Printed in Hong Kong by C & C Joint Printing Co (HK) Ltd

Will all the experience I acquired
Ever since my day of birth
Necessarily perish with me
When I leave this earth!

(ARAB POET, NINTH CENTURY AD)

This book is dedicated to the medical students and prac-
titioners who, it is hoped, will benefit from the author's lifelong
experience in the teaching and practice of gynaecological
diagnosis.

Preface

To see is to believe. This applies nowhere more accurately than in the teaching of clinical gynaecology. Yet because of the very nature of the subject, the ever increasing number of medical students and the paucity of clinical material, especially in the newer and smaller teaching hospitals, the demonstration of physical signs in clinical gynaecology is becoming exceedingly difficult and sometimes, in certain clinical entities, virtually impossible. Present day students of the subject generally hear too much and see too little.

There are a number of good books and monographs dealing with different aspects of clinical gynaecology. In most the text is satisfactory but the illustrations leave much to be desired. These considerations, plus my personal interest in photography, have prompted me to adopt a novel approach to explaining the principles of gynaecological diagnosis. Almost all important gynaecological symptoms and signs are described and their clinical significance discussed, but the text is presented in as concise a form as possible, and extensive use is made of colour photography to demonstrate the important diagnostic criteria. Because there are already several superbly illustrated works on gynaecological pathology, this part of the subject has not been touched upon.

The Kasr El Aini hospital is the oldest and largest teaching hospital in the Middle East and is a Mecca for interesting and difficult cases, both common and uncommon, in all medical specialties. It has taken some continuous hard work over the past 10 years to collect the material for this volume. Without the kindness and generosity of my colleagues who allowed access to their patients this work would not have been possible. I am especially grateful to the teaching staff, the clinical demonstrators and the resident doctors of my Section who have given tireless help and criticism.

All the colour photographs were made by me from cases in our Department, with the exception of Figures 4.71–4.75 which were kindly presented by Dr Michel Cognat of Lyon, France. The ultrasonography pictures (Figures 4.76–4.84) were made for me, also from our patients, by my assistant Dr A El Halafawi. To both of them I should like to express my thanks.

I also wish to thank my publishers for the excellent form in which they have produced this book.

Cairo, 1984   Abdel Fattah Youssef

Contents

1. Diseases of the Vulva   **1**

Congenital   2
Mechanical   4
Dystrophy. Skin affections. Inflammation. Ulcers   9
Cysts   27
Benign solid tumours   37
Malignant tumours   43
Urethral diseases   53

2. Diseases of the Vagina   **59**

Congenital   60
Mechanical conditions. Ulcers. Inflammation   68
Cysts   72
Benign tumours   78
Malignant tumours   80

3. Genital Prolapse   **85**

Types of prolapse. Degrees of uterine prolapse   86
Associated conditions. Complications   93
Recurrent prolapse   101

4. Perineal Tears. Rectovaginal Fistula.
     Genitourinary Fistulas   **103**

Perineal tears   104
Rectovaginal fistula   108
Genitourinary fistulas   110

5. Diseases of the Cervix Uteri   **119**

Congenital. Mechanical. Inflammation   120
Cervical erosion   125
Cervical polyp   130
Benign tumours   135
Carcinoma   138
Colposcopy   144

6. Diseases of the Corpus Uteri and the Adnexa   **149**

Fibroid polyp. Chronic inversion   150
Some other diseases of the corpus and the adnexa   157
Laparoscopy   166
Ultrasonography   168
Hysterosalpingography   171

References   **175**

Index   **177**

1. Diseases of the Vulva

Inspection plays a most important part in diagnosis of diseases of the vulva; hence the scope given to this topic in this illustrated treatise on gynaecological diagnosis.

Examination of the external genitals should always precede vaginal and bimanual examination. This should include examination of the vulva itself (labia minora, labia majora and clitoris) as well as inspection of the urethral opening, the vaginal introitus, the perineum and the anus. The patient should always be asked to strain with the labia separated as described later in the chapter on genital prolapse.

Since the vulva is mostly covered by skin, it is not surprising that many diseases of this organ lie so much in the domain of the dermatologist as in that of the gynaecologist. Inflammation, ulceration and dystrophy are examples of conditions in which both specialists should be equally interested. It is also noteworthy that the gynaecologist or the dermatologist may be the first to suspect, after simple inspection of the vulva, the presence of important related diseases. Examples are pruritus and monliasis which may be the first manifestations of diabetes, and Behçet's ulcers of the vulva which may be the clue to the dignosis of the neurological and/or occular complications of the Behçet syndrome.

On the other hand swellings of the vulva are a purely gynaecological problem. They are generally classified into:

1. Cystic swellings. These are always benign and are mostly of non-neoplasic origin. The Bartholin cyst, due to obstruction of the Bartholin duct, the inclusion epidermoid cyst, the hymenal cyst which originates from Wolfian relics in the hymenal region and the sebaceous cyst are the most important.

2. Solid swellings of the vulva are mostly neoplastic and may be benign or malignant.

(a) Benign vulval tumours of epithelial origin include the adenoma, hidradenoma and 'true' papilloma. They are all, as a rule, small in size. The papilloma is of considerable pathological interest since, histológically, it is closely related to the papillomata of inflammatory origin namely bilharzial papillomata and condylomata acuminata. Benign connective tissue tumours include the fibroma and lipoma which may reach a very large size. Angioma of the vulva is exceedingly rare.

(b) Malignant vulval tumours include epithelioma (by far the commonest), basal cell carcinoma (rodent ulcer), sarcoma, melanoma and choriocarcinoma. Basal cell carcinoma is always primary, choriocarcinoma is always metastatic. Epithelioma, sarcoma and melanoma of the vulva are usually primary but may be secondary.

Since inspection of the external urethral orifice should always be a part of examination of the external genitals, diseases of the urethra which may be detected by such inspection are included in this chapter.

Congenital

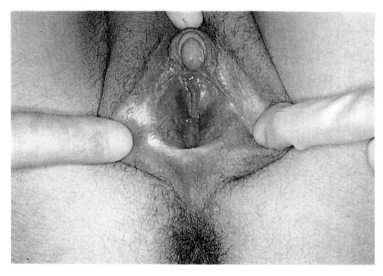

1.1

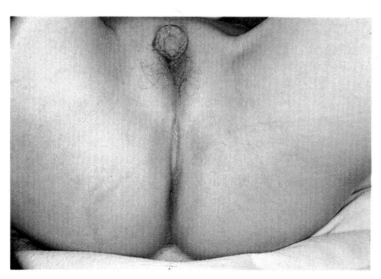

1.2

Figs 1.1–1.5 Intersexuality. Hypertrophy of Clitoris.
Hypertrophy of the clitoris is the commonest congenital abnormality of the vulva. It may be present alone (Fig. 1.1) or may be associated with labioscrotal fusion (Figs 1.2–1.4). The commonest cause of these anomalies is congenital adrenal hyperplasia but they may be due to other causes such as the ingestion of androgen during pregnancy or the association of an androgenic tumour with pregnancy. Adrenal hyperplasia is differentiated from other causes by the marked elevation of the 17-ketosteroid level in urine.

The presence or absence of labial fusion with the clitoral hypertrophy depends on the time of exposure of the female fetus to the androgenic effect. Labial fusion should be differentiated from labial adhesions (Figs 1.7–1.9) which are thought to be of inflammatory origin. In the latter condition there is no clitoral hypertrophy and no other manifestations of virilisation.

Fig. 1.5 shows a less common anomaly. The clitoris is hypertrophied (not seen in the picture), there is no labial fusion, but the gonads are present in the labia majora. Biopsy of these showed ovarian structure and the buccal smear was positive. This was therefore a case of female pseudohermaphroditism.

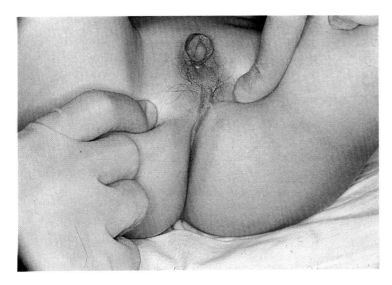

1.3

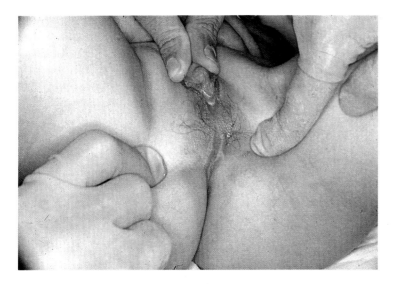

1.4

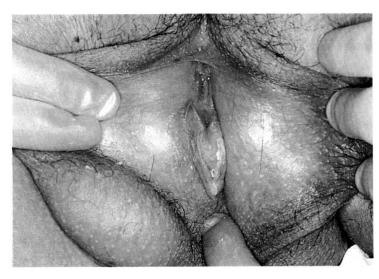

1.5

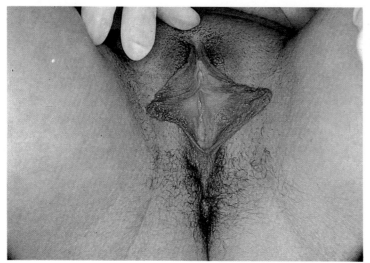

1.6

Fig. 1.6 Congenital Hypertrophy and Elongation of the Labia Minora. This usually causes no symptoms, but sometimes the patient complains of problems with personal hygiene, of friction during walking or of discomfort during sexual intercourse. She may also be worried by the cosmetic appearance.

Mechanical

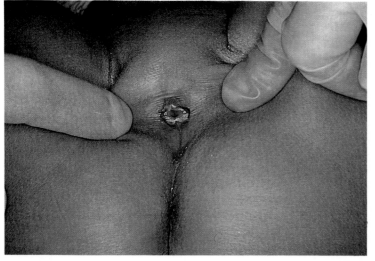

1.7

Figs 1.7–1.9 Labial Adhesions (Synechia vulvae) in infancy caused by low grade infection associated with hypo-oestrinism. The clitoris, vulva and genitals are normally developed. This should be differentiated from congenital labial fusion associated with hypertrophy of the clitoris (Figs 1.2–1.4). The child usually presents with urinary symptoms due to involvement of the urethral opening. Local treatment with oestrogen cream causes prompt separation of the adhesions.

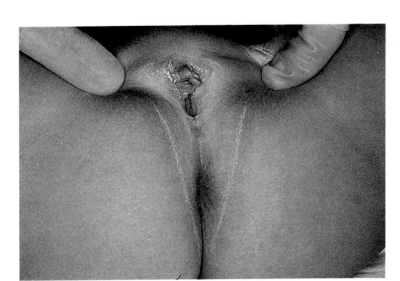

1.8

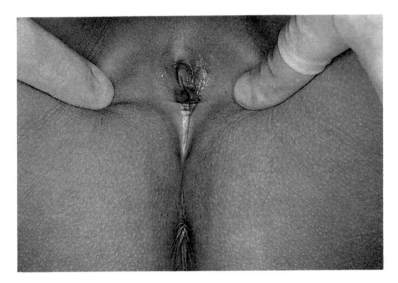

1.9

Fig. 1.10 Post-traumatic Labial Adhesions Following Accidental Injury.

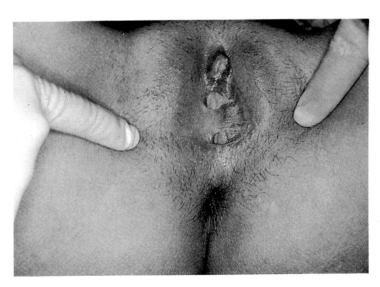

1.10

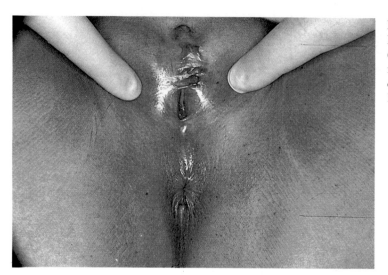

1.11

Figs 1.11–1.13 Post-traumatic Labial Adhesions Following Circumcision. They may be diffuse (Fig. 1.11) or band-like (Figs 1.12 and 1.13). They may be symptomless or the patient may complain of dyspareunia. They are frequently torn during labour.

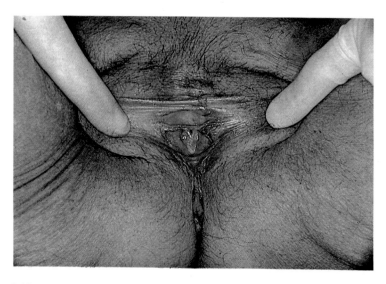

1.12

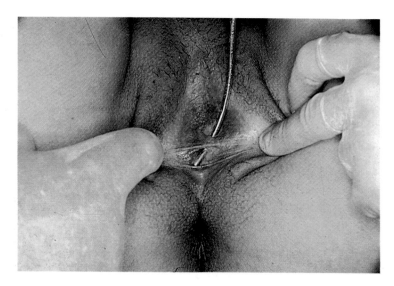

1.13

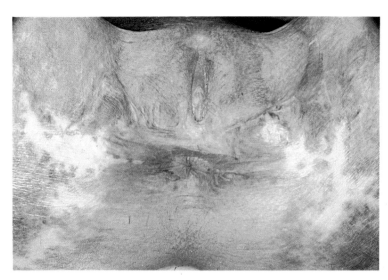

1.14

Figs 1.14 & 1.15 Post-traumatic Labial Adhesions Following Burn. Marked disfiguring and almost complete closure of the vestibule. The patient complained of difficulty and pain during intercourse.

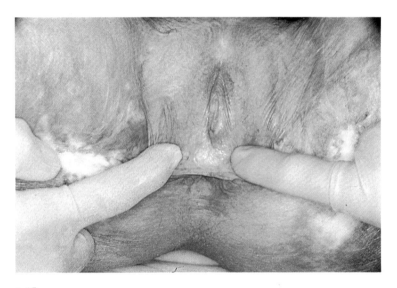

1.15

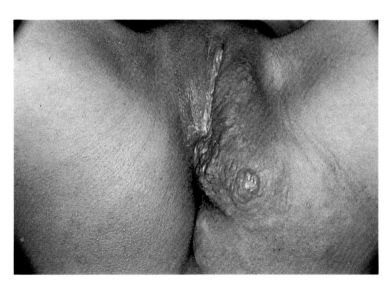

1.16

Figs 1.16 & 1.17 Varicosities of the Vulva. The vulval veins on the left side in Fig. 1.16 and on the right side in Fig. 1.17 are enlarged and tortuous giving rise to a bulging compressible bluish swelling. Palpation discloses the worm-like sensation of the varicose veins. The symptoms are swelling and discomfort especially on standing or walking. Possible complications are haemorrhage and thrombosis.

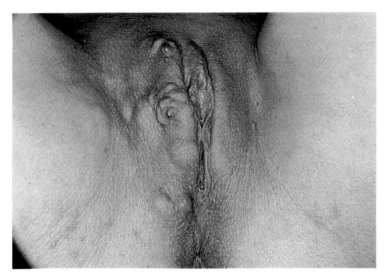

1.17

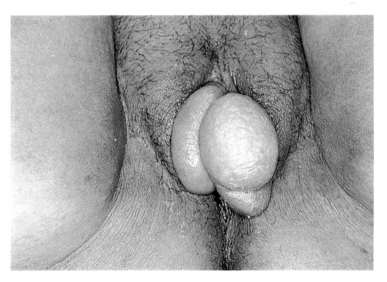

1.18

Fig. 1.18 Oedema of the Vulva. Marked oedema of both labia minora in this case was due to pre-eclampsia. In addition to symptoms of pre-eclampsia the patient complained of swelling and discomfort in the vulval region. Pitting on pressure could be demonstrated. Unlike in inflammatory oedema (Figs 1.38, 1.39 and 1.85) there was no tenderness, warmth or redness of the affected parts.

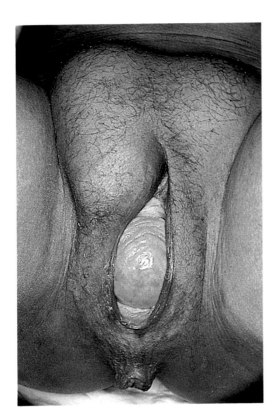

1.19

Fig. 1.19 Bilateral Inguinal Hernia. Cystocele. Piles. The hernia is more marked on the right side and protrudes into the upper part of the labium majus on either side. The swellings were soft, reducible and had an expansile impulse on coughing.

Dystrophy–Skin affections– Inflammation–Ulcers

Leukoplakia signifies the presence of thickened elevated white patches in the skin of the vulva, often complicated by fissuring and ulceration. The patient complains of intense itching and the lesion may be precancerous.

The International Society for the Study of Vulval Disease has recently proposed the use of the term 'hyperplastic dystrophy' instead of leuko-plakia.[1] It has also suggested that cases of hyperplastic dystrophy be classi-fied into those without and those with atypia and maintained that only the latter may be precancerous. Undoubtedly this is a useful pathological classi-fication which has a bearing on prognosis and treatment.

However, 'leukoplakia' is a well established clinically descriptive term which is still used by clinicians of exceptional experience.[2] It is therefore considered appropriate to use it in this atlas.

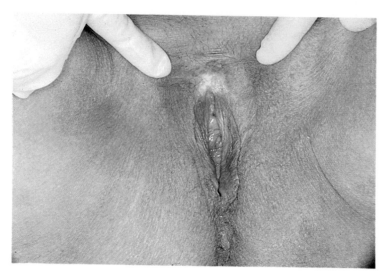

1.20

Fig. 1.20 Leukoplakia. Localized thickened elevated white patches around clitoris.

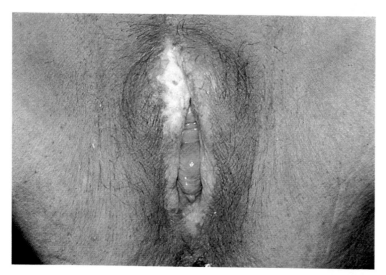

1.21

Fig. 1.21 Leukoplakia. Here the labia minora are also involved. The lesion is much more marked in the anterior part of the vulva where it probably started.

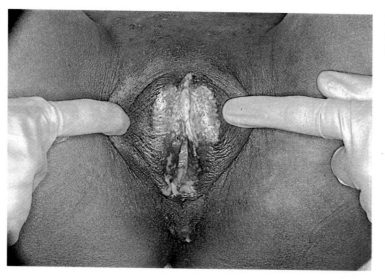

1.22

Fig. 1.22 Leukoplakia. Occasionally the disease affects the inner aspects of the labia minora with little involvement of the clitoral region.

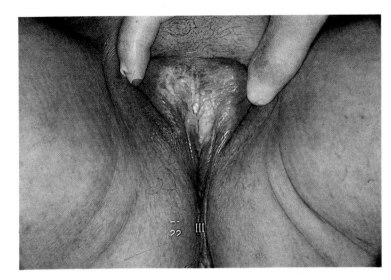

1.23

Fig. 1.23 Leukoplakia. Fissuring has appeared in the anterior part of the vulva especially in the right side.

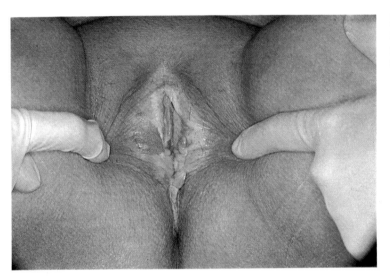

1.24

Fig. 1.24 Leukoplakia. A large superficial ulcer is seen in the inner surface of the right labium majus. Serial sectioning showed atypia but no malignancy.

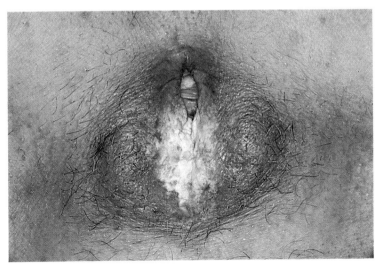

1.25

Fig. 1.25 Leukoplakia. Markedly thickened elevated well delineated pearly white appearance. Note that even in extensive leukoplakia the process does not involve the outer aspects of the labia majora or the perianal region.

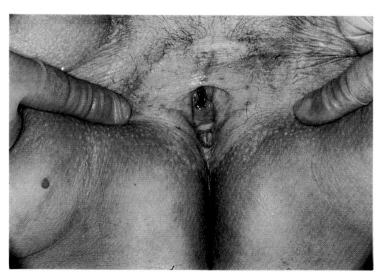

1.26

Figs 1.26 & 1.27 Lichen Sclerosus. Smooth waxen parchment-like shrunken appearance of skin of vulva and perineum. Loss of subcutaneous fat. Narrowing of the introitus. The condition, formerly often called 'kraurosis', represents the atrophic type of vulval dystrophy.

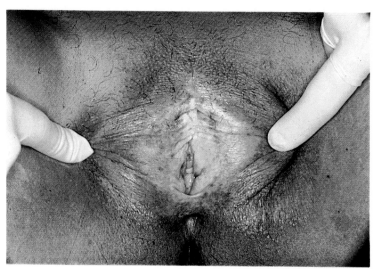

1.27

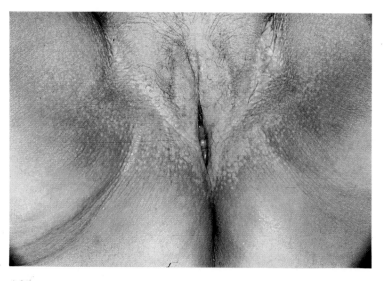

1.28

Fig. 1.28 Lichen Planus. The vestibule and inner aspects of the labia show the characteristic delicate bluish white atrophic appearance. Very small pruplish papules are seen.

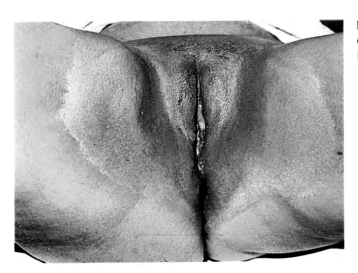

Fig. 1.29 Intertrigo. Skin affection due to friction of contiguous surfaces. Colour at first red, fades into various shades of grey.

1.29

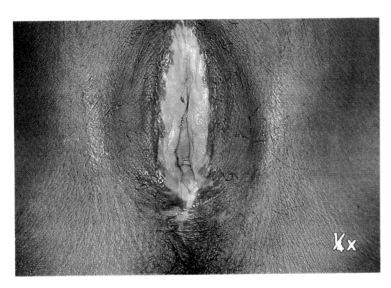

Figs 1.30–1.36 Leukoderma. Depigmentation in sharply defined areas of skin and/or mucous membranes. No thickening, elevation, fissuring or ulceration ever occur. The condition most commonly affects the inner surfaces of the labia majora and minora (Figs 1.30–1.34) but it may also be present in the clitoral region (Fig. 1.35). Unlike leukoplakia, it may also involve the outer aspects of the labia majora and even the skin outside the vulva (Fig. 1.36). The depigmentation has a more striking appearance in dark coloured patients (Figs 1.33 and 1.34). The condition is not associated with any particular symptoms.

1.30

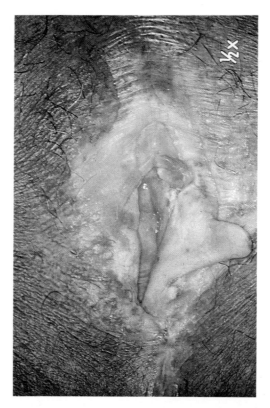

1.31

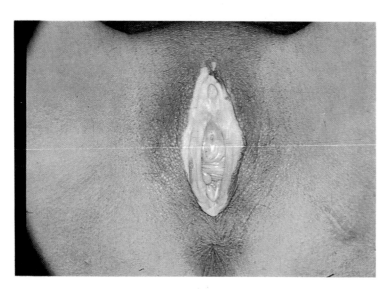

1.32

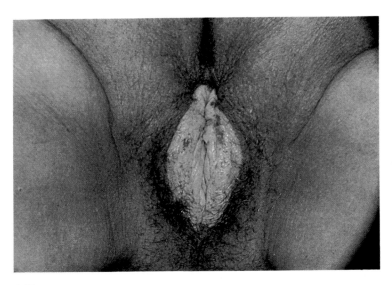

1.33

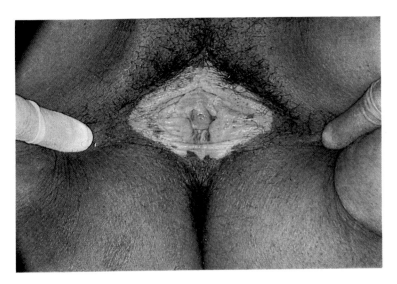

1.34

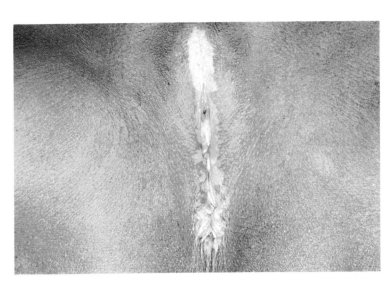

1.35

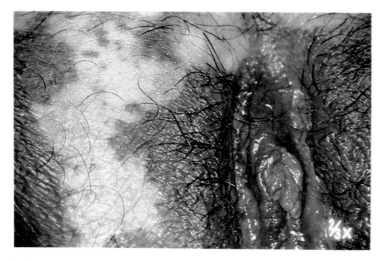

1.36

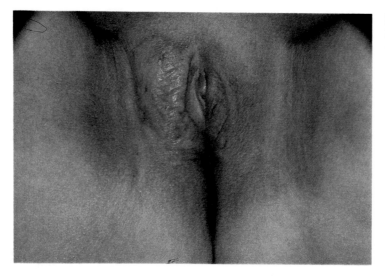

1.37

Fig. 1.37 Allergic Dermatitis of Right Labium Majus. Erythema, oedema and ulceration are visible. The vagina is always spared.

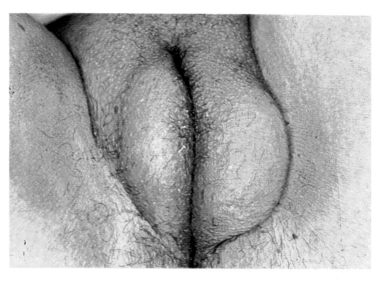

1.38

Fig. 1.38 Acute Nonspecific Vulvitis. Redness and oedema of both labia majora.

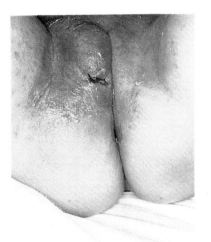

Fig. 1.39 Acute Nonspecific Vulvitis. Abscess of right labium majus has complicated an infected wound.

1.39

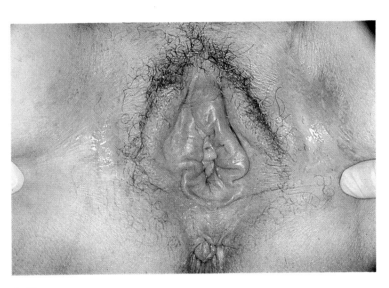

Figs 1.40–1.44 Monilia Vulvitis. These cases illustrate the 10 typical features recently described by Gardner and Kaufman:[3] 1. Extensive involvement of the perianal skin, inner thighs and mons. 2. Oedema. 3. Erythema (livid colour, beefy, bright or intensely red). 4. Thrush patches. 5. Superficial greyish white film, sometimes giving boiled or cooked appearance, sometimes a reddish blue hue. 6. Glazed shining appearance of skin. 7. Satellite vesicopustules. 8. Excoriations from scratching and fissuring in the skin's natural folds. 9. Depigmentation in dark complexioned patients. 10. Furunculosis of vulval skin.

1.40

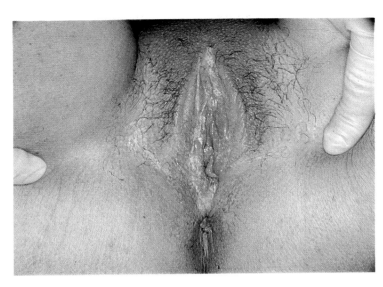

1.41

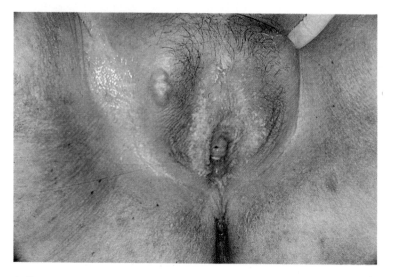

1.42

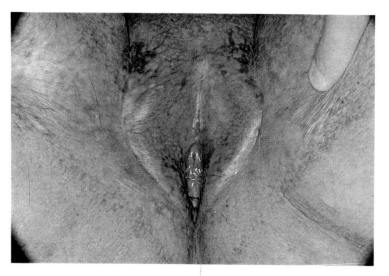

1.43

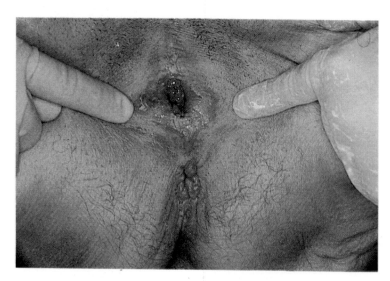

1.44

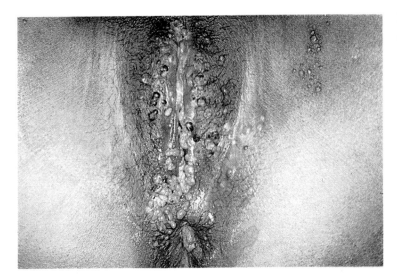

Fig. 1.45 Condylomata Acuminata. Multiple greyish or pinkish warts scattered on both labia.

1.45

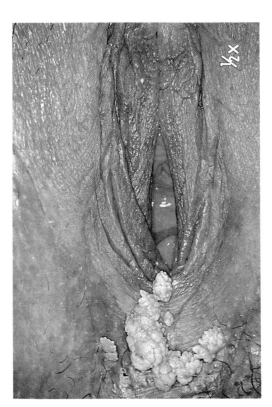

Fig. 1.46 Condylomata Acuminata. In this case the lesions are confluent forming fleshy masses especially in the perineum and perianal region.

1.46

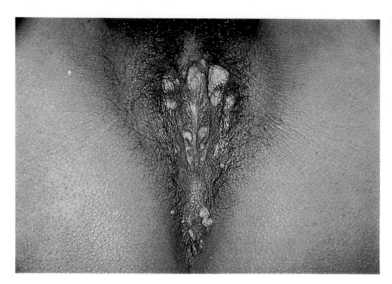

Fig. 1.47 Condylomata Lata. Raised white plaques covered by serous exudate in vulva, perineum and perianal region.

1.47

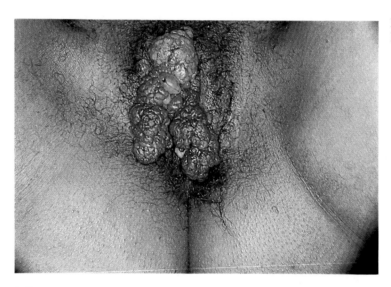

Figs 1.48 & 1.49 Multiple Large Bilharzial Papillomata affecting both labia majora.

1.48

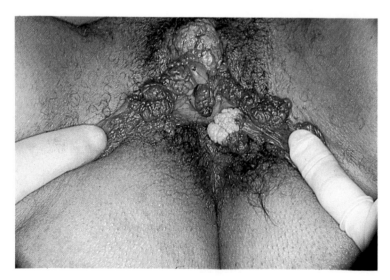

1.49

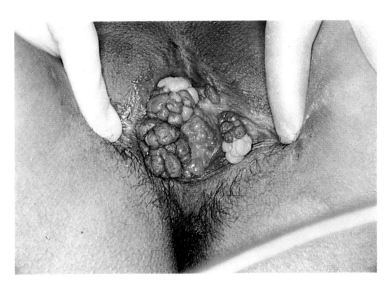

Fig. 1.50 Bilharzial Papillomata affecting labia majora. The lesion is more advanced on the right side.

1.50

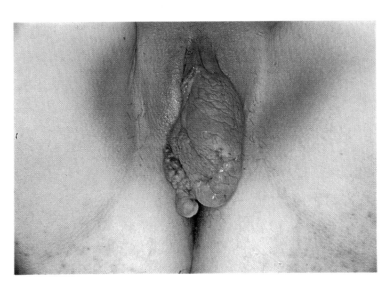

Figs 1.51 & 1.52 Large Bilharzial Mass of the left labium majus. Separation of the labia demonstrates the typical papillomata.

1.51

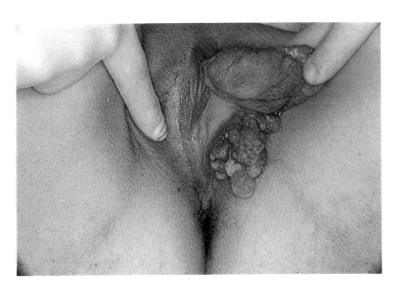

1.52

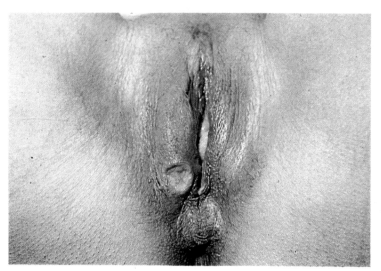

1.53

Figs 1.53 & 1.54 Behçet's Syndrome. Simultaneous ulceration of vulva and mouth. The vulval ulcer on the right labium majus has the typical appearance described by Behçet: round, a few centimetres in diameter, with a smooth yellowish base. The mouth ulcer affects the right cheek. This young girl also had iridocyclitis.

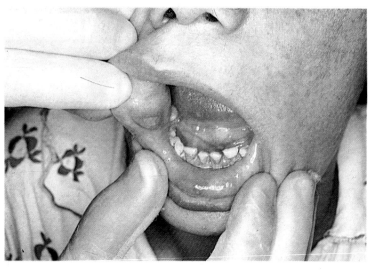

1.54

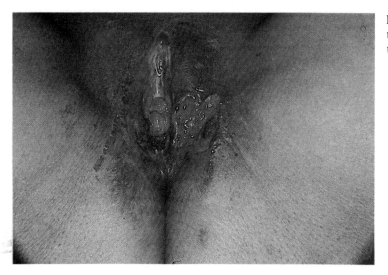

1.55

Figs 1.55 & 1.56 Behçet's Syndrome. Simultaneous ulceration of the vulva and mouth. In this case the mouth ulcer affects the lower lip.

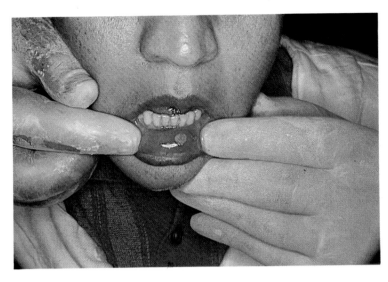

1.56

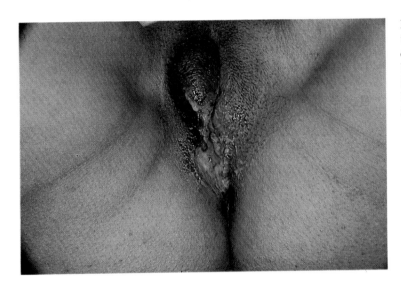

Fig. 1.57 Granuloma Inguinale. Ulcer charac-
teristically spreading toward perineum has raised
edges, serpentine in outline, and a raw red base.
Note the characteristic hypertrophy and oedema,
in this case affecting the right labium majus.
Donovan bodies were demonstrated confirming
the diagnosis.

1.57

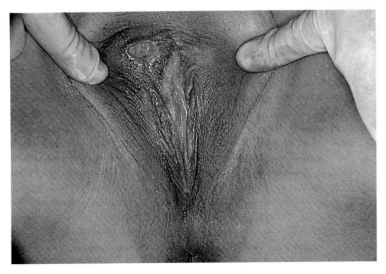

Fig. 1.58 Syphilis. Primary sore seen in the
upper part of the right labium majus. Note the
characteristic punched out appearance, circular
shape and shiny glistening surface. There was
marked inguinal lymphadenitis. Treponema
pallidum was demonstrated in smear.

1.58

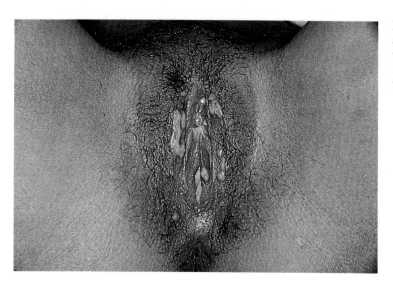

1.59

Figs 1.59–1.61 Herpes Simplex. Lesions mainly affecting the labial skin. In Fig. 1.59 the small vesicles are almost all intact. In Figs 1.60 and 1.61 some vesicles have broken down giving rise to shallow ulcers.

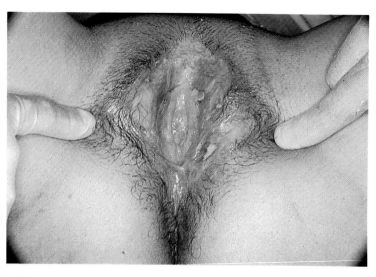

1.60

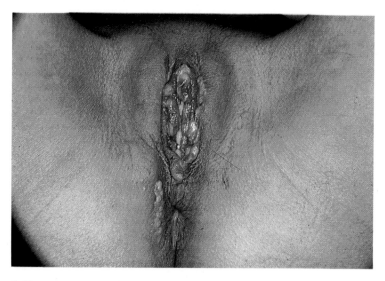

1.61

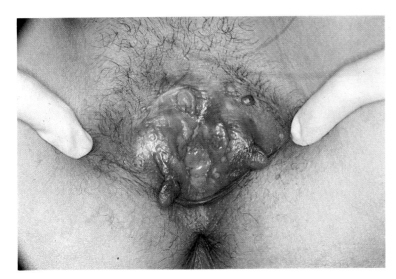

1.62

Figs 1.62 & 1.63 Herpes Simplex. Lesions mainly affecting the mucosa at the vestibule. In Fig. 1.62 some vesicles are intact, some are ulcerated. In Fig. 1.63 a single ulcer resulting from the breakdown of multiple neighbouring vesicles is present anteriorly in the inner surface of the right labium minus.

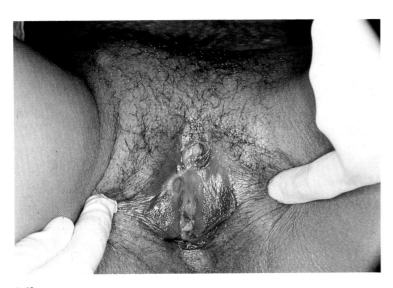

1.63

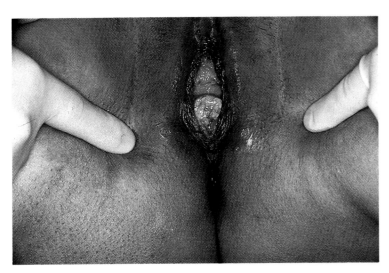

1.64

Fig. 1.64 Nonspecific Inflammatory Ulcers. Superficial ulcers with dirty yellowish base complicating furunculosis of the vulva resulting from dribbling of urine in a case of urinary incontinence.

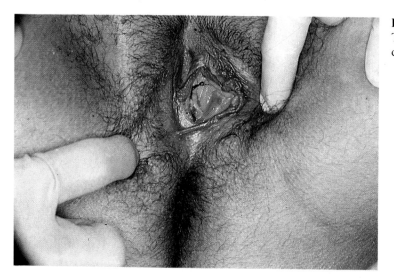

Figs 1.65 and 1.66 Infected Traumatic Ulcers.
The ulcer in Fig. 1.65 resulted from injury by a douche nozzle.

1.65

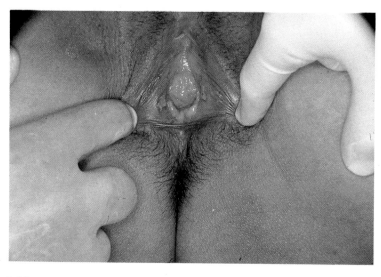

1.66

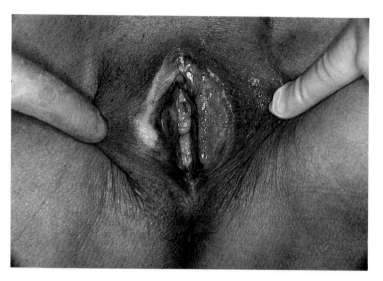

Fig. 1.67 Allergic Ulcer. Large superficial ulcer of left labium majus following the use of a local antiseptic lotion.

1.67

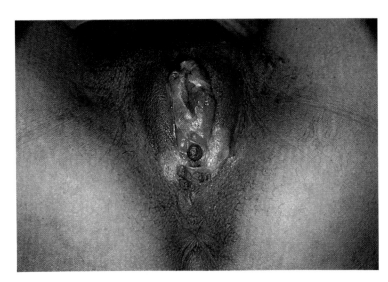

Fig. 1.68 Allergic Ulcers. Oedema and extensive ulceration of the vulva following the application of a topical antibiotic ointment.

1.68

Cysts

Cysts of the vulva may be symptomless or the patient may complain of dyspareunia and/or a vulval swelling. If they become infected the symptoms of inflammation are superimposed.

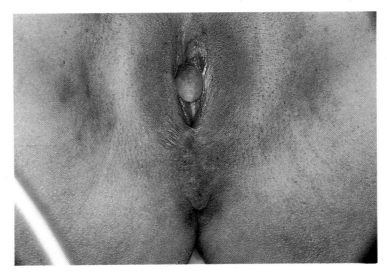

Figs 1.69–1.76 Epidermoid Cyst. In female circumcision parts of the clitoris and the two labia minora are excised. Epidermal inclusion cysts are not uncommon following this procedure. They vary in size from small (Fig. 1.69) to fairly large (Fig. 1.72). In Figs 1.69–1.72 the cyst is unilocular. In Figs 1.69 and 1.70 the cyst is related to the clitoral stump; in Fig. 1.71 it is attached to the stump of the right labium minus, while in Fig. 1.72 the cyst is too large to allow determination of its exact origin.

In Figs 1.73–1.76 the cyst is bilocular. In Fig. 1.73 the two locules are related to the clitoral stump. In Fig. 1.74 a cyst is present in each labium minus. In the case illustrated in Figs 1.75 and 1.76 a cyst is present in relation to the clitoral remnant and a smaller one in relation to the remnant of the left labium minus.

1.69

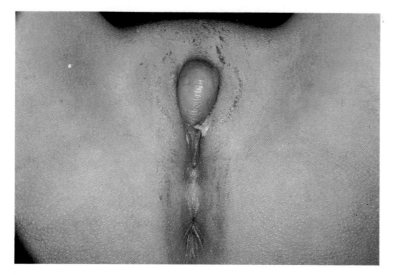

1.70

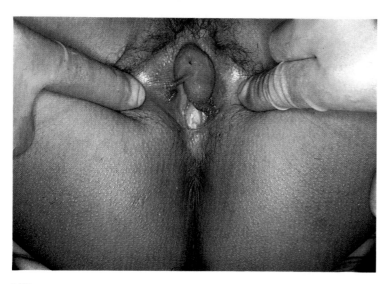

1.71

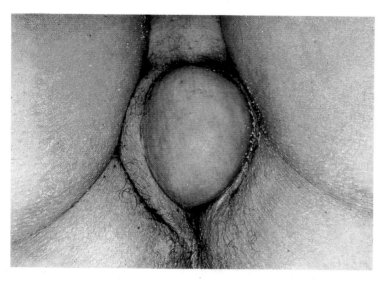

1.72

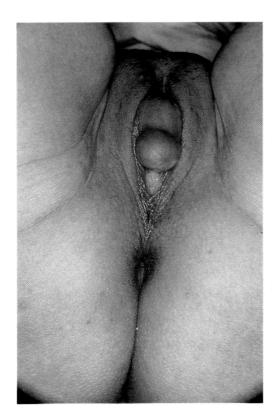

1.73

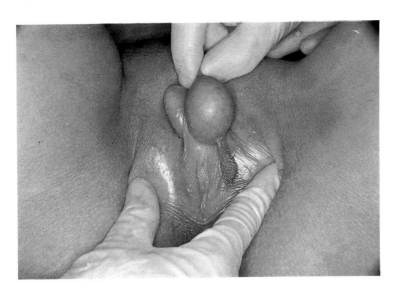

1.74

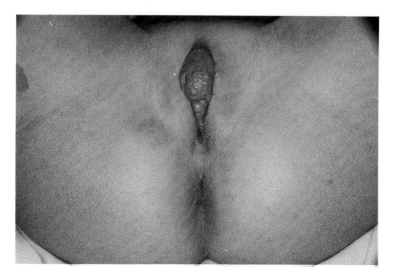

1.75

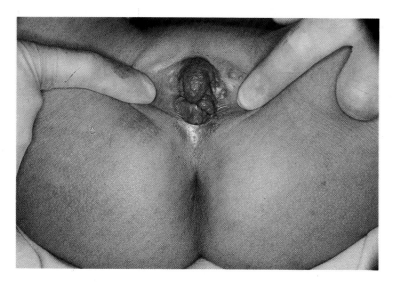

1.76

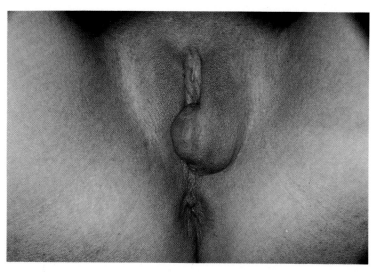

1.77

Figs 1.77–1.85 Bartholin Cyst. Caused by obstruction of the Bartholin duct, this common cyst of the vulva occupies the site of the Bartholin gland in the posterior part of the labium majus. The site of the cystic swelling points to the diagnosis (Figs 1.77–1.83). The site and shape of the cyst often result in the characteristic S shape of the vaginal introitus (Figs 1.79, 1.81). The swelling is often pyriform in shape with the base toward the anus and the apex toward the pubis (Figs 1.78, 1.80, 1.82). If the labia are separated, the labium minus is seen to be stretched over the cyst (Figs 1.78, 1.80, 1.82, 1.83).

The cyst is usually only a few centimetres in diameter, but may become much larger (Figs 1.83, 1.84) especially when infection gives rise to Bartholin abscess, whereupon the the swelling becomes tense, very painful and tender and there may be redness and oedema of the skin (Fig. 1.85).

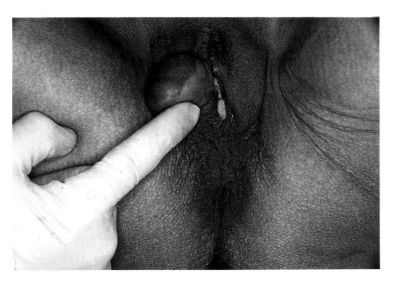

1.78

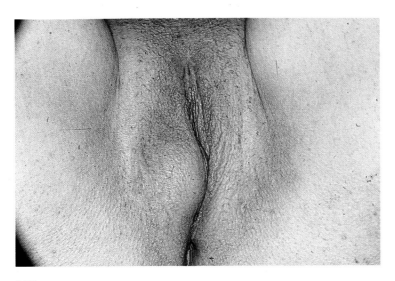

1.79

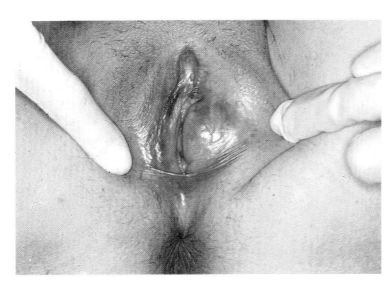

1.80

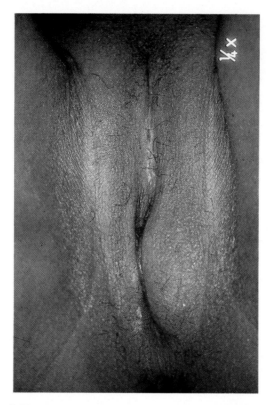

1.81

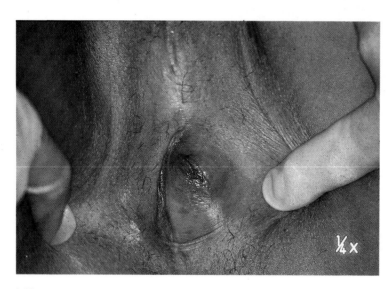

1.82

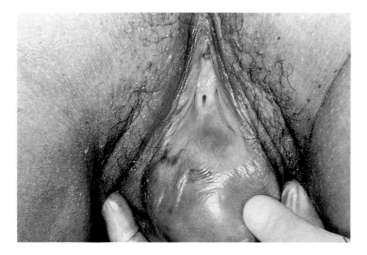

1.83

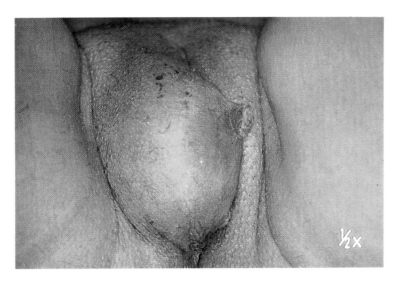

1.84

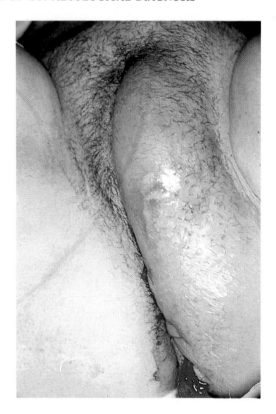

1.85

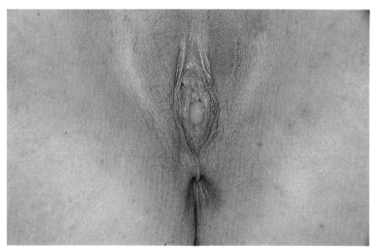

1.86

Figs 1.86–1.88 Hymenal Cyst. Small cysts of congenital origin seen within the vestibule close to the caruncula myrtiformis. May arise from remnants of the mesonephros, like similar vaginal and cervical cysts, or of the urogenital sinus. May be single (Figs 1.86, 1.87) or multiple (Fig. 1.88).

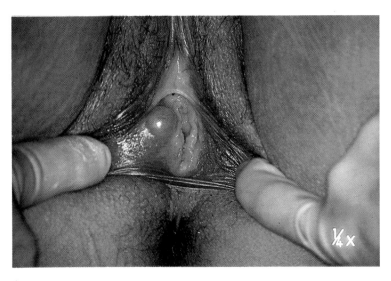

1.87

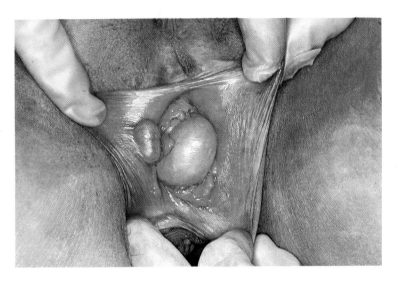

1.88

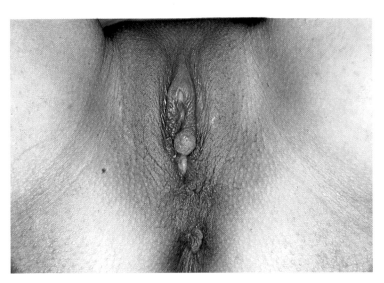

1.89

Figs 1.89–1.92 Sebaceous Cyst. Small cysts caused by blockage of the ducts of sebaceous glands contain characteristic cheesy material. May arisé in the labia majora or in the labia minora.

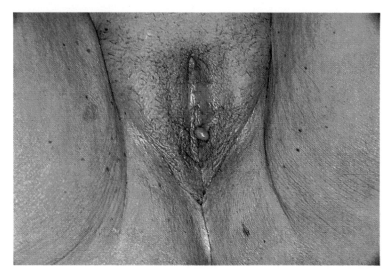

1.90

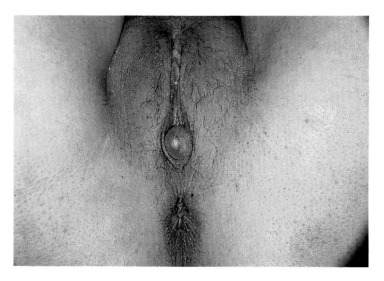

1.91

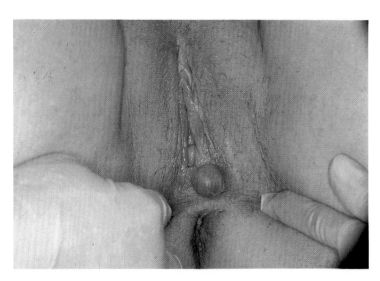

1.92

Benign solid tumours

Benign solid tumours of the vulva may cause no symptoms or the patient may complain of dyspareunia and/or a vulval swelling. Occasionally the tumour may reach such a large size as to cause discomfort on sitting or walking.

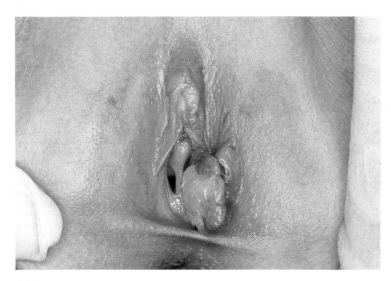

Figs 1.93–1.96 True Papilloma. Warty sessile growth arises most usually from labium majus (Figs 1.93–1.95), less commonly from labium minus (Fig. 1.96). Differentiated from Bilharzial papillomata and condylomata acuminata by being always single.

1.93

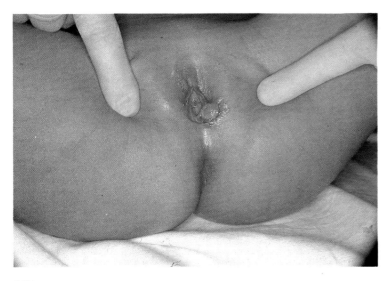

1.94

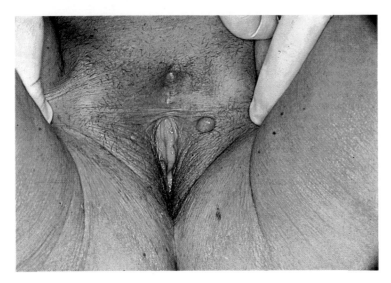

1.95

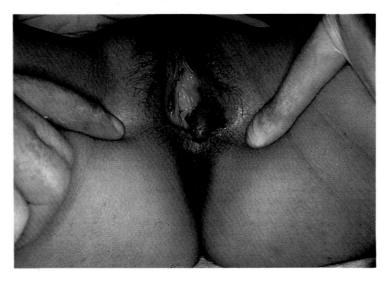

1.96

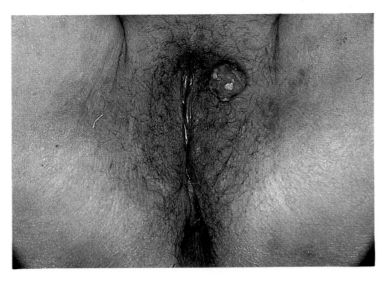

1.97

Fig. 1.97 Hidradenoma. Well circumscribed, slightly elevated lesion; the skin covering it is ulcerated and granular. Arises from the apocrine glands and is always situated in the labium majus.

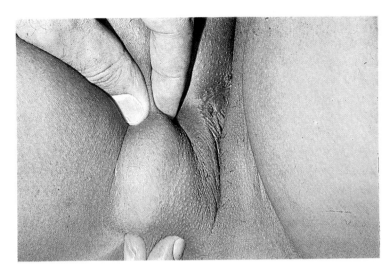

Fig. 1.98 Lipoma. Soft lobulated tumour arising in right labium majus.

1.98

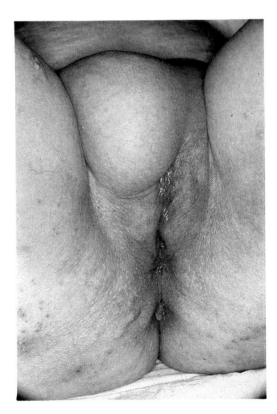

Figs. 1.99 Lipoma. Arising in mons pubis and growing into upper part of right labium majus.

1.99

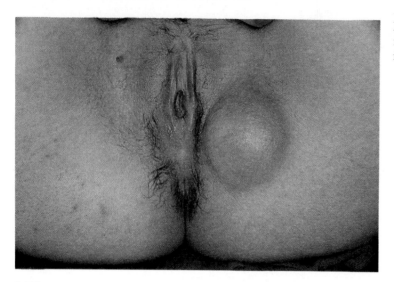

1.100

Fig. 1.100 Lipoma. Soft lobulated tumour arising in the fatty tissue of the buttock and growing into lower part of left labium majus.

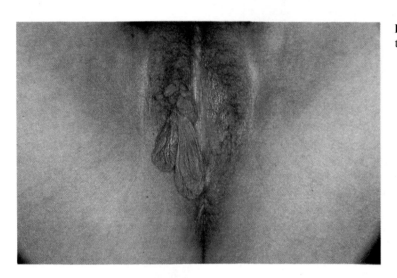

1.101

Figs. 1.101 & 1.102 Fibroma. Pedunculated tumour arising from right labium majus.

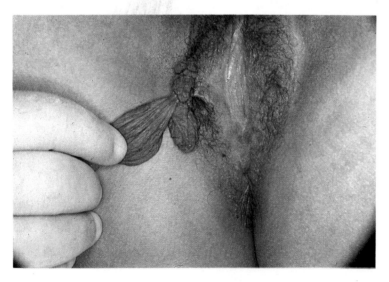

1.102

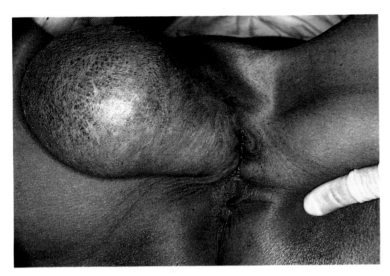

Fig. 1.103 Fibroma. A huge more or less sessile tumour arising from right labium majus.

1.103

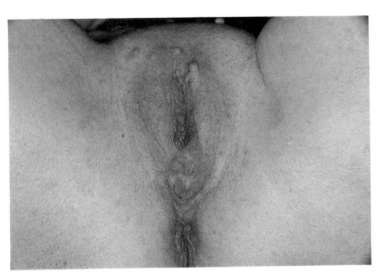

Figs 1.104 & 1.105 Multiple Neurofibromatosis (von Recklinghausen's Disease). Fig. 1.104: small firm discrete greyish nodules in the vulva. Fig. 1.105: similar lesions scattered all over the body.

1.104

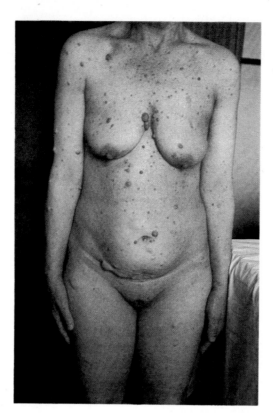

1.105

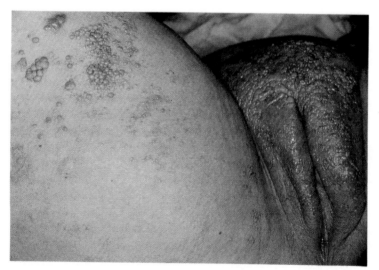

1.106

Figs 1.106 & 1.107 Lymphangioma Circumscriptum. Affecting the vulva and the medial aspect of the right thigh. In this case the lesion is rather extensive. Note the small deep vesicles, some of which contain blood. In the vulva they are closely aggregated, in the thigh more diffuse.

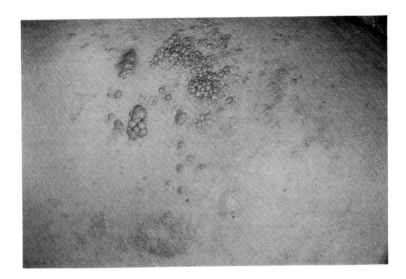

1.107

Malignant tumours

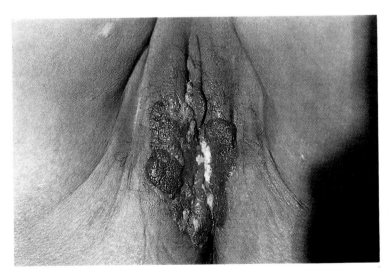

Fig. 1.108 Bowen's Disease. Small leukoplakic patches with superficial ulceration of the left labium majus associated with intense pruritus. Biopsy revealed carcinoma *in situ*.

1.108

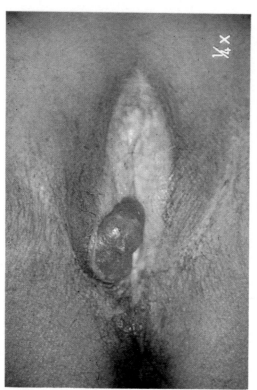

1.109

The ulcer may be on level with the adjacent skin (Fig. 1.111) or it may be elevated with everted edges (Fig. 1.109). Leukoplakia, sometimes quite marked, can be associated with carcinoma and may be its precursor (Figs 1.109, 1.114).

Figs 1.109–1.115 Epithelioma (Endophytic or Ulcerative Type). When the ulcer is present on the outer surface of the labium majus (Figs 1.109–1.111) the lesion is usually unilateral. When the ulcerative lesion affects the inner aspects of the labia and the vestibule the lesion is usually bilateral and symmetrical, the so-called kissing ulcers (Figs 1.112–1.115).

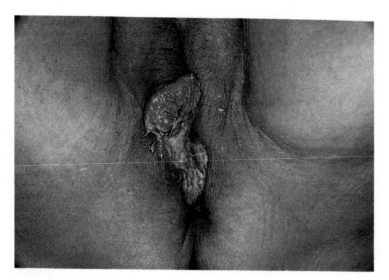

1.110

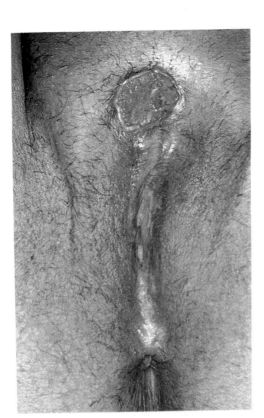

1.111

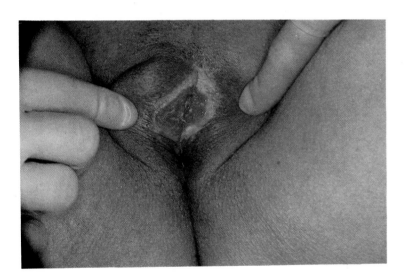

1.112

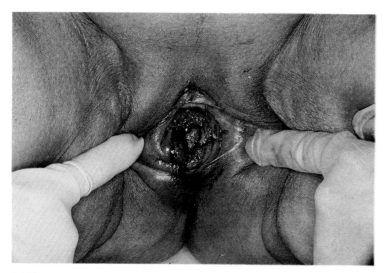

1.113

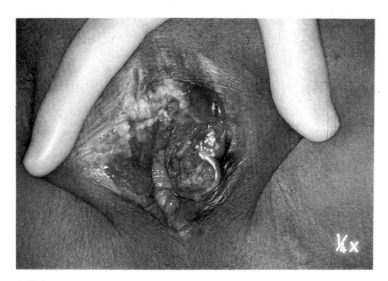

1.114

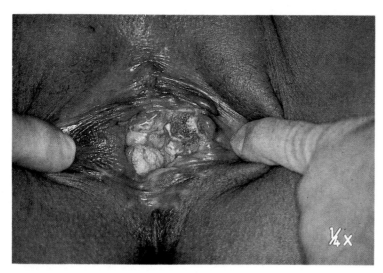

1.115

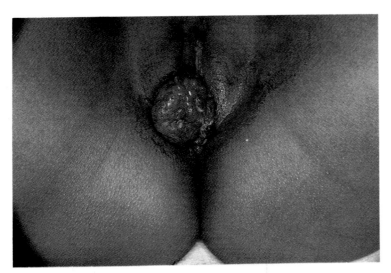

1.116

Figs 1.116–1.121 Epithelioma (Exophytic or Fungoid Type). This most commonly arises in the labium majus and is almost always initially unilateral and may remain so even when fairly advanced (Figs 1.116–1.119). Sometimes it spreads to the contralateral side, usually across the introitus or the perineum (Figs 1.120, 1.121).

The fungating growth almost always undergoes ulceration although this may be slight and occur at a late stage. Oedema of the vulva may be pronounced (Figs 1.118, 1.119). Leukoplakia may be associated (Figs 1.120, 1.121), but is less common and usually less marked than in the ulcerative type.

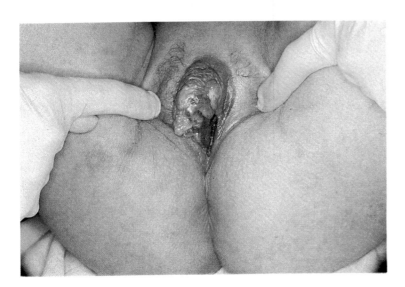

1.117

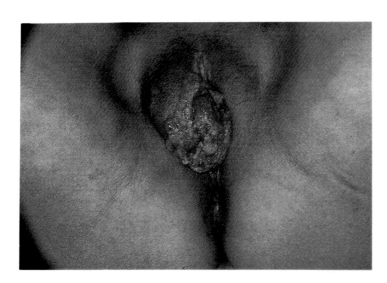

1.118

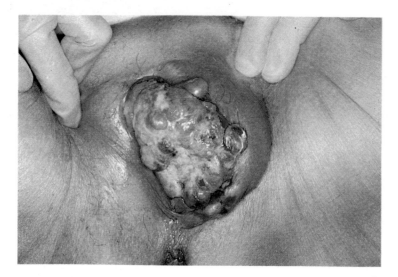

1.119

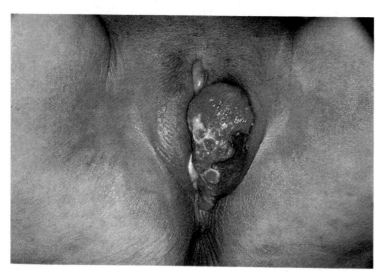

1.120

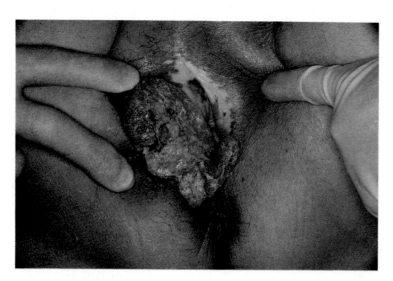

1.121

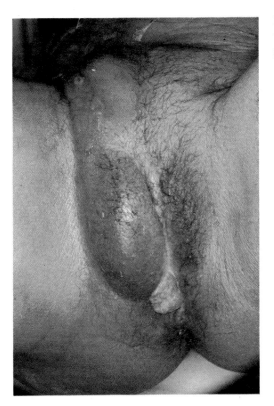

Figs 1.122 & 1.123 Epithelioma of Vulva with visible involvement and breakdown of the inguinal lymph nodes.

1.122

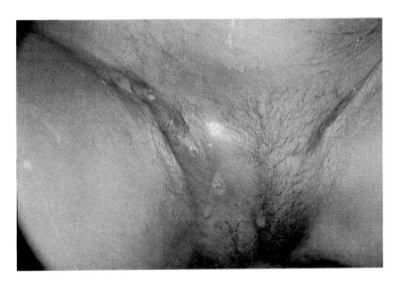

1.123

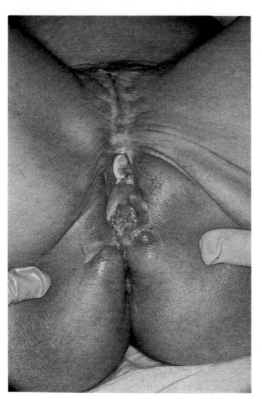

1.124

Fig. 1.124 Recurrent Epithelioma. Small ulcer in posterior end of radical vulvectomy scar.

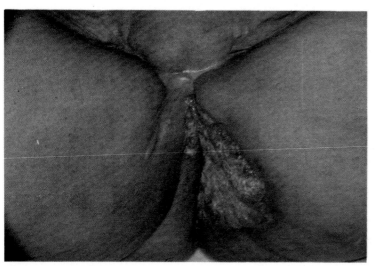

1.125

Fig. 1.125 Recurrent Epithelioma (Endophytic Type). Large elevated ulcer with everted edges infiltrating scar, perineum and left groin.

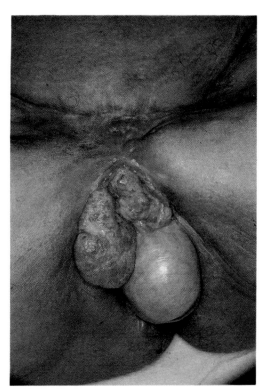

Figs 1.126 & 1.127 Recurrent Epithelioma (Exophytic Type). Fungating growth in region of mons pubis and right groin also infiltrating urethra and upper vagina. Associated second degree uterine prolapse. The prolapse antedated the recurrence in this elderly patient and may be due in part to the division of the pelvic floor muscles in the radical vulvectomy.

1.126

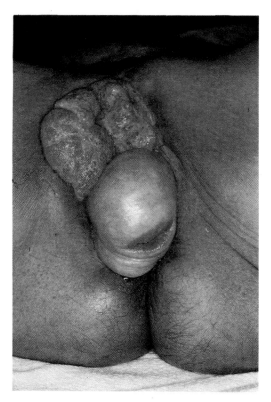

1.127

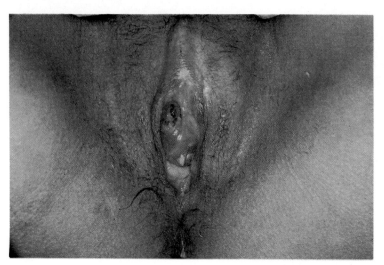

1.128

Figs 1.128–1.130 Choriocarcinoma (Metastatic).
Figs 1.128, 1.129: dark bluish raised nodule in the
anterolateral part of the vestibule just outside the
hymenal tags. Fig. 1.130: similar nodules in the
thigh. The patient also had uterine bleeding and
haemoptysis which suggested the right diagnosis.
This was confirmed by high HCG titre and
biopsy.

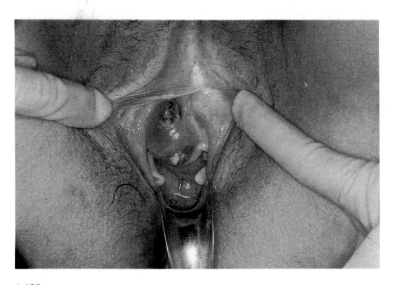

1.129

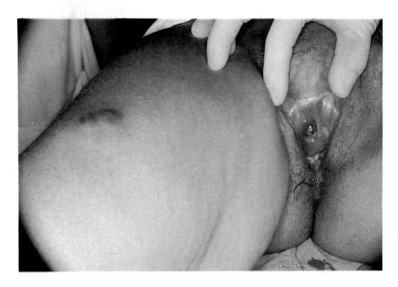

1.130

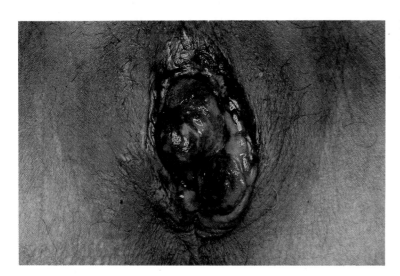

Fig. 1.131 Malignant Melanoma. Elevated pigmented very dark brown growths of the vulva infiltrating the lower vagina.

1.131

Urethral diseases

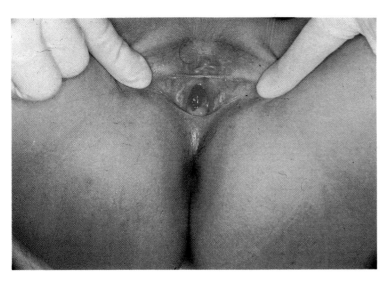

Figs 1.132–1.135 Urethral Caruncle. Reddish polypoid swelling, size of a pea, attached to the posterior lip of the meatus and protruding externally. Figs 1.133, 1.135 show catheter introduced into the urethra in the same cases as in Figs 1.132 and 1.134 respectively.

1.132

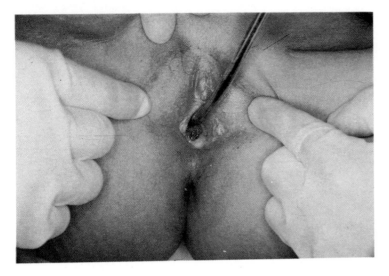

1.133

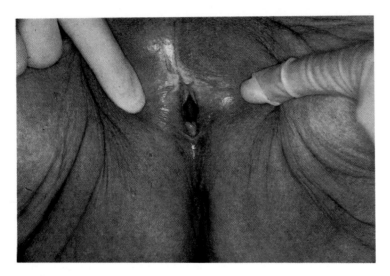

1.134

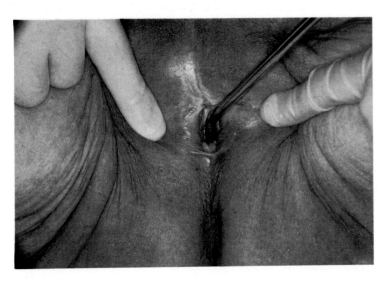

1.135

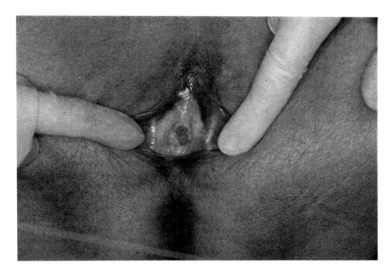

1.136

Fig. 1.136 Urethral Caruncle. Although caruncles are usually single (Figs 1.132–1.135), two or more caruncles may be present. In this case two caruncles are seen attached to the posterior lip of the urethral meatus.

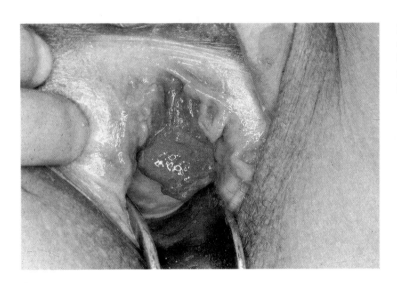

1.137

Figs 1.137 & 1.138 Urethral Caruncle. This caruncle is very unusual in that it is much larger in size than usual and is seen to arise from the anterior lip of the meatus. Histological examination showed it to be bilharzial.

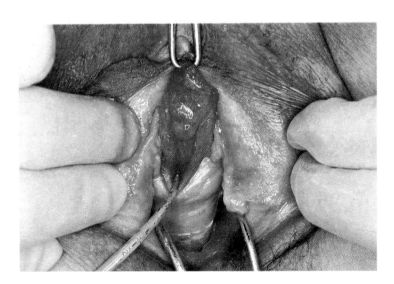

1.138

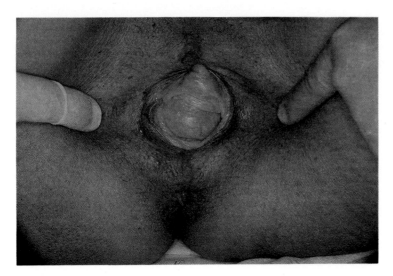

1.139

Figs 1.139 & 1.140 Cyst of the Urethra. Arising from Skene's glands. A rare condition.

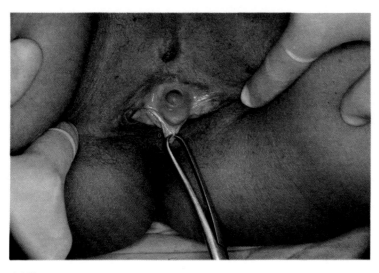

1.140

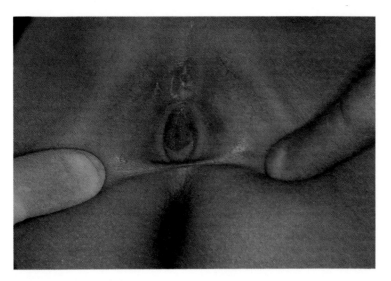

1.141

Figs 1.141–1.143 Prolapse of the Urethra. A deep red annular swelling protrudes from and replaces the meatus. The fact that the whole circumference of the urethra is affected differentiates it from urethral caruncle. Fig. 1.143 shows a catheter introduced into the urethra in the same case as in Fig. 1.142.

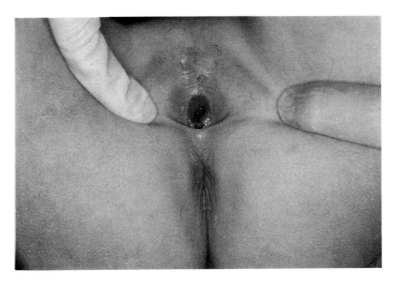

1.142

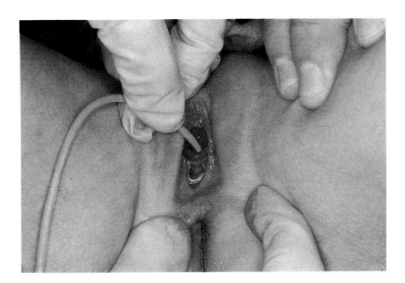

1.143

Figs 1.144 & 1.145 Carcinoma of the Urethra.
Polypoid infiltrating mass arising from inside the
urethra with no relation to the vulva.

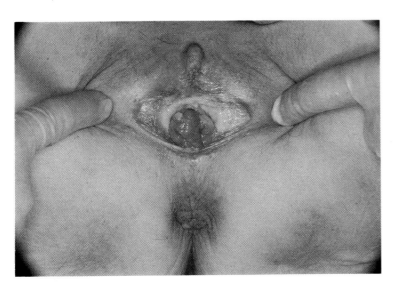

1.144

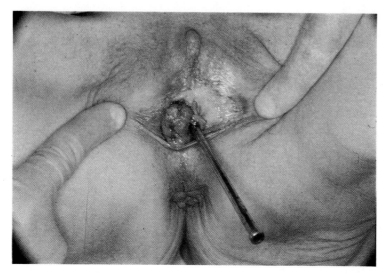

1.145

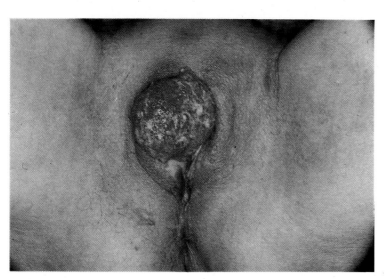

1.146

Fig. 1.146 Vulvourethral Carcinoma. A fungating mass with extensive infiltration of the lower half of urethra and clitoral region. The origin of the tumour, whether urethral or vulval, is not possible to determine. Biopsy showed moderately differentiated squamous cell carcinoma.

2. Diseases of the Vagina

The vagina and the cervix are the only internal genital organs amenable to inspection, albeit with the use of special specula and retractors. Diseases of these organs can thus be visually demonstrated and directly photographed and are therefore adequately covered in this volume.

Certain congenital conditions of the vagina such as duplication, longitudinal and transverse septa can often be better seen than felt. It is surprising how often such abnormalities are completely missed by the casual examiner. In all cases of congenital anomalies of the genital tract intravenous pyelography should be carried out, for association of urinary tract anomalies is not uncommon.

Common inflammations of the vagina such as those caused by monilia and trichomonas infection are usually associated with similar inflammation of the vulva and/or cervix.

The only important cysts of the vagina are the Gaertner cyst and the epidermoid cyst and they are of the same origin as the hymenal and epidermoid cysts of the vulva respectively.

Tumours of the vagina are less common than those of any female genital organ with the exception of the Fallopian tube.

Carcinoma is the commonest malignant tumour of the vagina but is relatively much less common than carcinoma of the cervix or vulva. It is therefore a rule in clinical gynaecology that the diagnosis of primary carcinoma of the vagina should only be made when the cervix and the vulva are not involved. In other words, if carcinoma of the vagina is associated with carcinoma of the cervix or vulva the tumour in the vagina should be considered as secondary. In recent years attention has been drawn to vaginal adenosis and neoplasia in cases exposed *in utero* to the administration of diethylstilboestrol.

Congenital

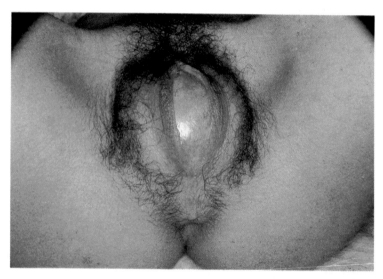

2.1

Figs 2.1–2.5 Haematocolpos. Cryptpmenorrhoea (false amenorrhoea) caused by an imperforate hymen or by a transverse vaginal septum just above the hymen. The vagina is distended with altered blood and the hymen bulges outwards. Depending on the thickness of the septum, it may appear bluish (Figs 2.1, 2.2) or may be of pale pink colour (Fig. 2.3).

Shortly after puberty the patient complains of cyclic lower abdominal colicky pains. The uterus is always pushed upwards and may also be distended with blood (haematometra) whereupon a suprapubic swelling will be seen and felt (Fig. 2.4). On incision of the obstructing septum the retained dark coloured blood is released (Fig. 2.5).

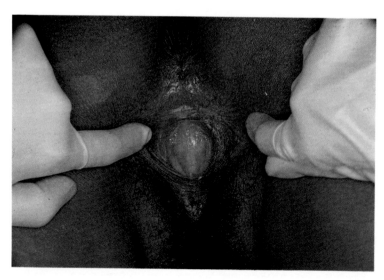

2.2

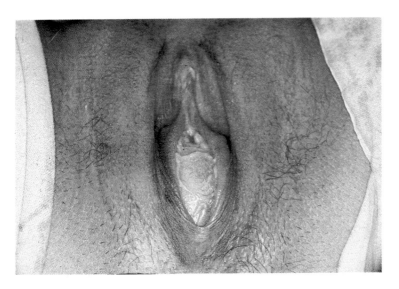

2.3

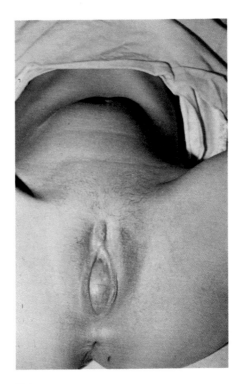

2.4

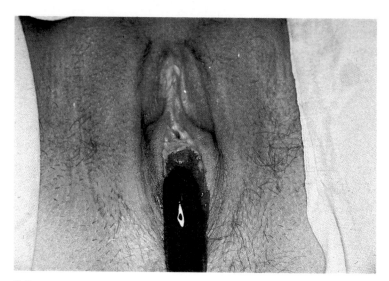

2.5

Figs 2.6–2.10 Aplasia of the Vagina. Congenital absence of the vagina results from incomplete development and canalization of the Muellerian ducts. It is usually associated with absence or gross underdevelopment of the uterus and primary amenorrhoea. The absence or rudimentary condition of the uterus can be diagnosed on rectal examination. Associated anomalies of the urinary tract are common and should be looked for.

The external genitals are normal and the vagina is represented by a small blind pouch developed from the urogenital sinus (Figs 2.6–2.8). Normal sexual intercourse is of course not possible and in some cases coitus per urethra is practised and the urethral orifice appears markedly dilated (Figs 2.9, 2.10).

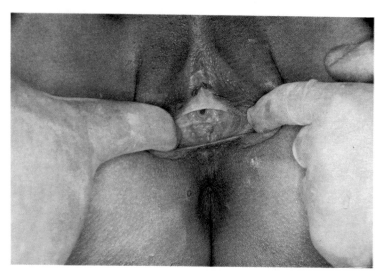

2.6

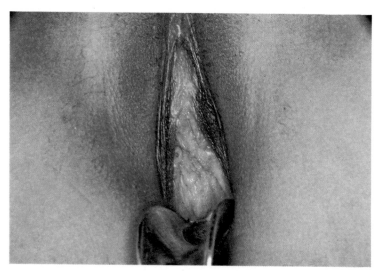

2.7

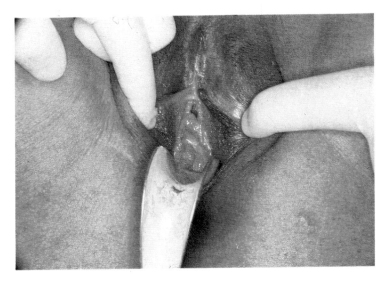

2.8

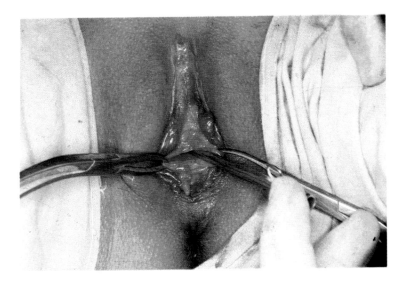

2.9

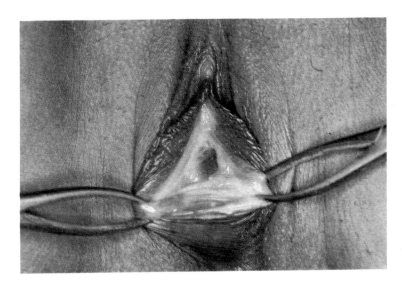

2.10

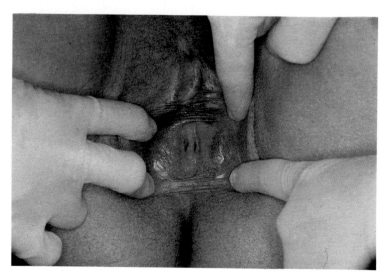

2.11

Figs 2.11 & 2.12 Longitudinal Vaginal Septum (Partial). In this case the septum was present only in the lower half of the vagina.

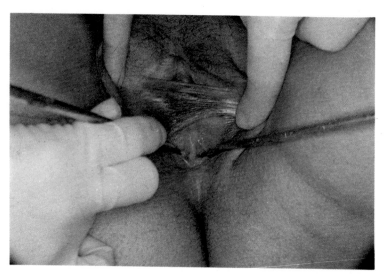

2.12

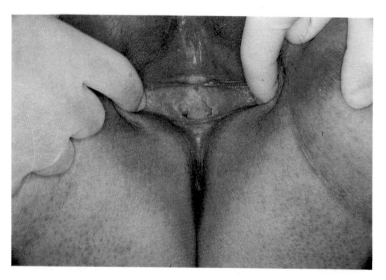

2.13

Figs 2.13 & 2.14 Longitudinal Vaginal Septum (Complete). In this case the longitudinal septum reached up to the cervix (double vagina). The extent of the septum can only be determined by vaginal examination.

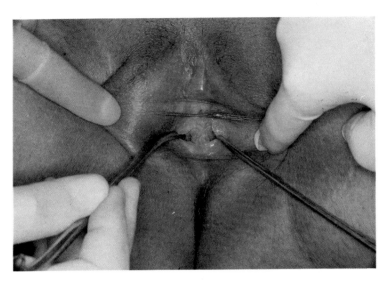

2.14

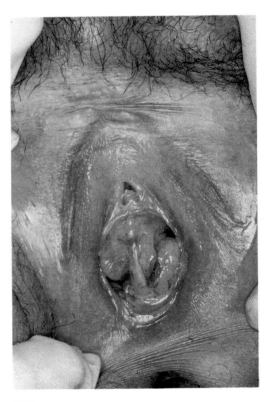

2.15

Fig. 2.15 Longitudinal Vaginal Septum (Complete). This patient had double vagina and also double cervix and double uterus (uterus pseudodidelphys). The tissues look oedematous because she had had a recent abortion.

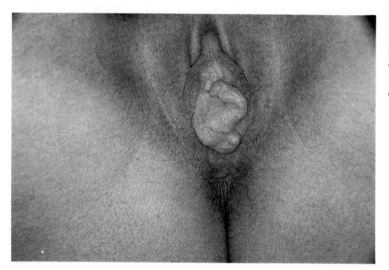

2.16

Figs 2.16 & 2.17 Longitudinal Vaginal Septum torn by previous delivery. This unusual condition can be mistaken by the inexperienced for tumour or prolapse. But, as can be seen in the illustration, no tumour is present and the genital organs are in their normal postion.

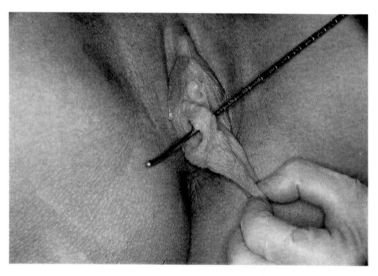

2.17

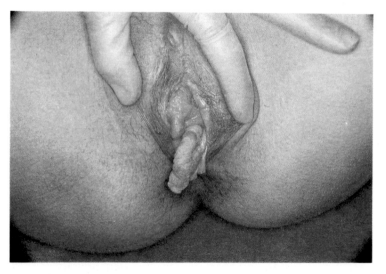

2.18

Figs 2.18 & 2.19 Longitudinal Vaginal Septum torn by previous delivery. Another example of this uncommon entity.

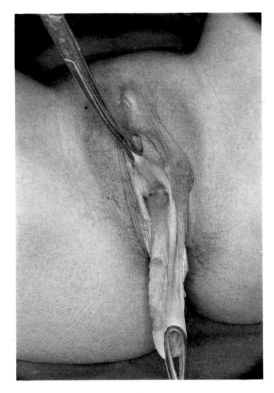

2.19

Mechanical conditions–
Ulcers–Inflammation

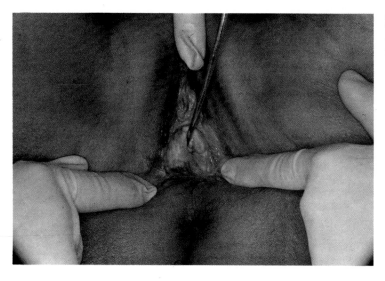

Fig. 2.20 Traumatic Atresia of the Vagina.
Almost complete atresia following inexperienced
surgical repair of cystorectocele.

2.20

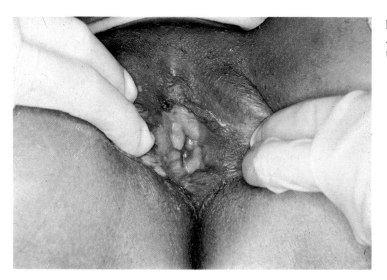

**Fig. 2.21 Traumatic Vaginal Atresia Following
Accidental Injury.** In such cases the chief symptoms are dyspareunia and infertility.

2.21

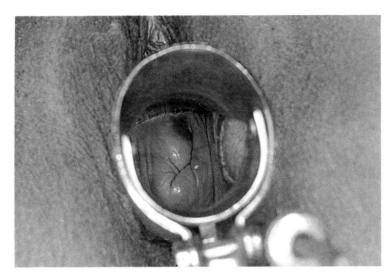

Fig. 2.22 Pigmentation of the Vagina. Dark brown areas for no apparent reason may be accidentally discovered on speculum examination. They give rise to no symptoms (For pigmentation in cases of genital prolapse see Figs 3.22 and 3.23.)

2.22

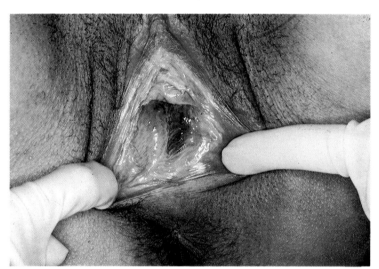

Fig. 2.23 Haematoma of Vagina. A dark purple firm tender vaginal swelling affecting mostly the left lateral vaginal wall. In this case the haematoma followed a spontaneous vaginal delivery.

2.23

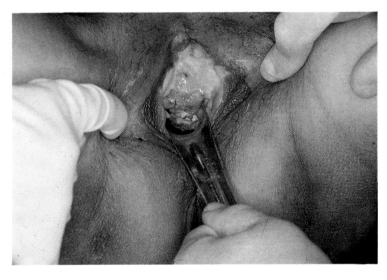

Fig. 2.24 Extensive Ulceration of the Vagina. In this case the ulceration followed the local use of an unknown medication for the treatment of infertility!

2.24

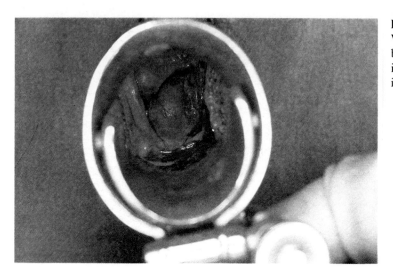

Fig. 2.25 Traumatic Ulcer of the Posterior Vaginal Wall following the insertion of a foreign body. The edges of the ulcer show no eversion or induration. This together with the absence of any infiltration attest to its benign nature.

2.25

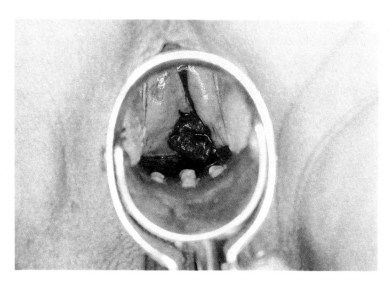

Fig. 2.26 Septic Granulation Tissue at the Vaginal Vault. This is a not uncommon cause of discharge and contact bleeding after total hysterectomy. Cytology and biopsy may be necessary to exclude malignancy. The condition is treated by diathermy coagulation under anaesthesia.

2.26

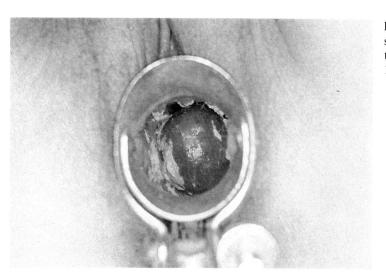

Fig. 2.27 Monilia Vaginitis. This is usually associated with monilial vulvitis and gives rise to the same symptoms and physical signs (see Figs 1.40–1.44).

2.27

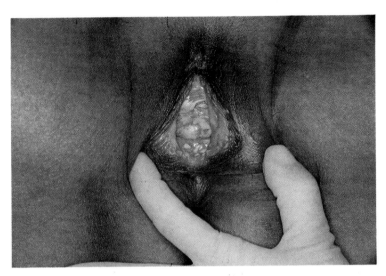

2.28

Fig. 2.28 Senile Vaginitis. Diffuse inflammation of the vaginal mucosa in an elderly patient with multiple small superficial ulcers. The chief complaints are dyspareunia and offensive blood stained discharge. If the latter symptom is present malignancy should always be looked for.

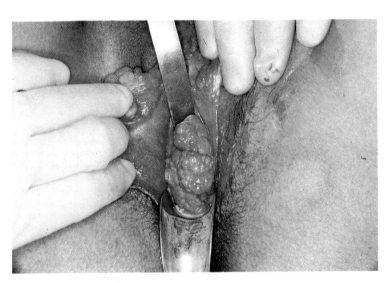

2.29

Figs 2.29–2.31 Bilharzial Papillomata of the Vagina. These may be apparent on external examination (Fig. 2.29) and may be assoicated with vulval papillomata. Smaller lesions, especially when situated high in the vagina may only be seen on speculum examination (Figs 2.30, 2.31).

Bilharzial papillomata are always multiple, vary in size and show no signs of iduration or infiltration. Secondary infection and bleeding on touch are much less marked than in vaginal malignancy, The diagnosis is established by cytology and biopsy. It is believed that the lesion may be precancerous (see Fig. 2.56).

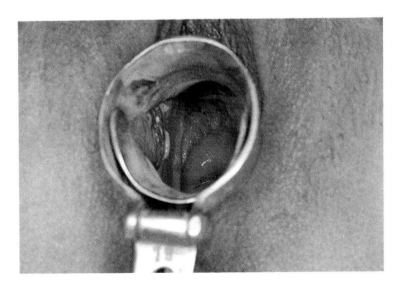

2.30

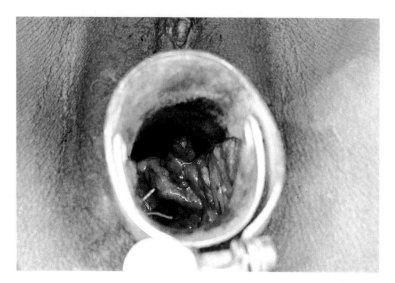

2.31

Cysts

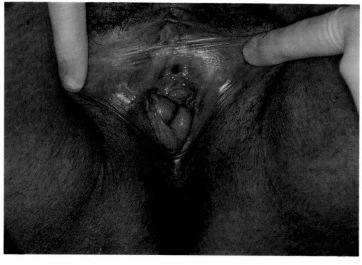

2.32

Figs 2.32–2.40 Gaertner Cysts of the Vagina.
These arise from vestigial remnants of the
Wolfian duct and are therefore always present in
the anterior or lateral vaginal walls. The illustrations show that they vary much in size.

They may be present low down in the vagina
(Figs 2.32, 2.33) and look much like hymenal
cysts (Figs 1.86–1.88) which are of similar origin,
but the vaginal cysts lie deeper inside the introitus. Or they may be present high up in the
vagina in the fornix or closely related to the
cervix (Fig. 2.34) in which cases the diagnosis
presents no difficulty. When of small size
Gaertner cysts of the vagina are thin walled and
have a characteristic bluish colour (Figs 2.32–
2.34).

Less commonly they reach a much larger size
and are then thick walled and frequently mis-

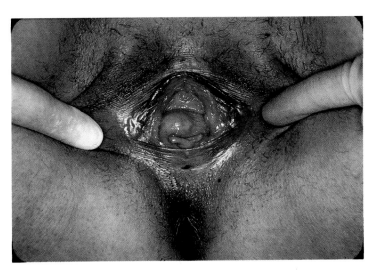

2.33

taken for cystocele. In the two similar cases
shown in Figs 2.35–2.37 and in Figs 2.38, 2.39
the patient presented with a mass protruding
from the vulva which was first thought to be a
cystocele (Figs 2.36, 2.38). On separation of the
labia (Figs 2.36, 2.38) and palpation of the swelling, it was found to be a well-defined irreducible
fluctuant cystic swelling which could not therefore be a cystocele. Pulling on the swelling (Figs
2.37, 2.39) shows its true relations to the vaginal
wall, and introducing a cathether into the urethra
(Fig. 2.39) shows that the bladder is in its normal
position and helps to establish the diagnosis. Fig.
2.40 shows one of the largest Gaertner cysts ever
seen by the author.

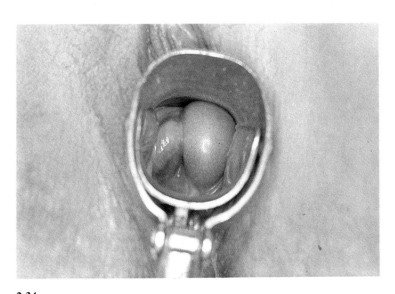

2.34

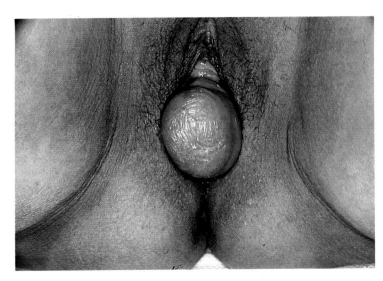

2.35

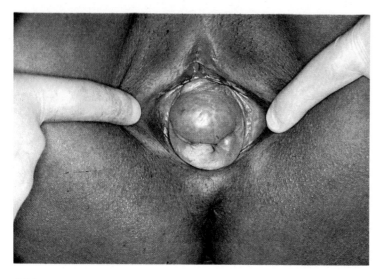

2.36

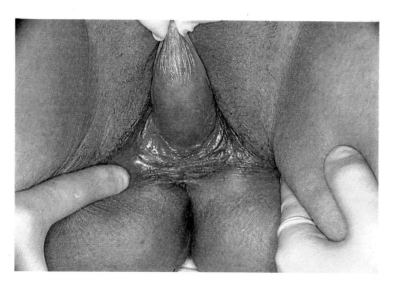

2.37

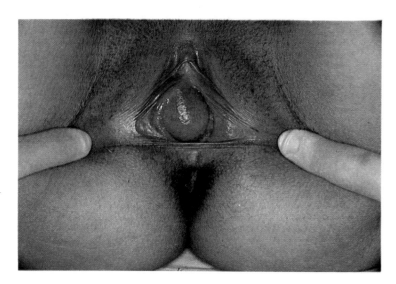

2.38

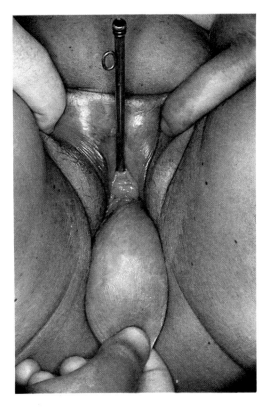

2.39

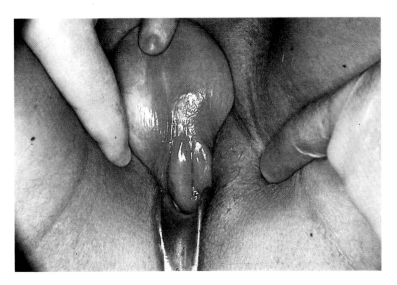

2.40

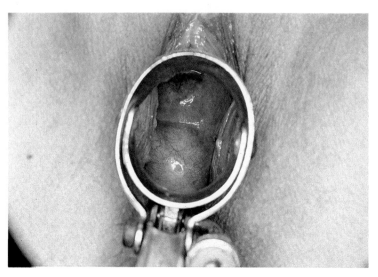

2.41

Figs 2.41–2.46 Cysts of the Posterior Vaginal Wall. These are less common and their origin less clear than the Gaertner cysts. It is believed that most of them are caused by inclusion of vaginal epithelium during labour or surgery. When situated high up in the vagina (Fig. 2.41), or in the middle vagina (Fig. 2.42) the diagnosis is obvious.

When present low down in the vagina and of big size (Figs 2.43–2.46) they may easily be mistaken for rectocele. The facts that they are irreducible and do not increase in size on straining point to their true nature. Separating the labia (Fig. 2.44) and pulling on the cyst (Figs 2.45, 2.46) help to show its relation to the posterior vaginal wall, and rectal examination should confirm the diagnosis.

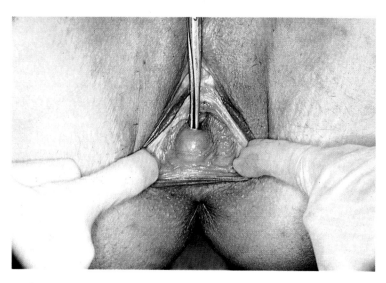

2.42

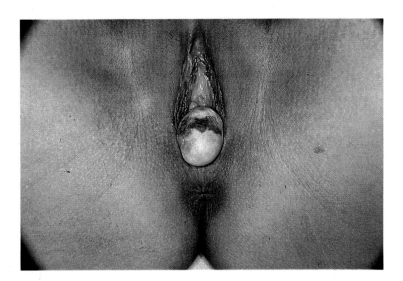

2.43

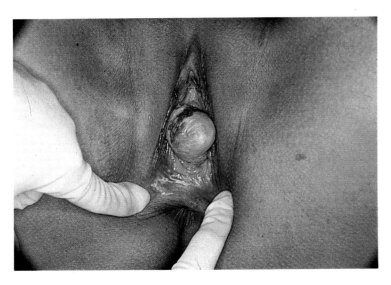

2.44

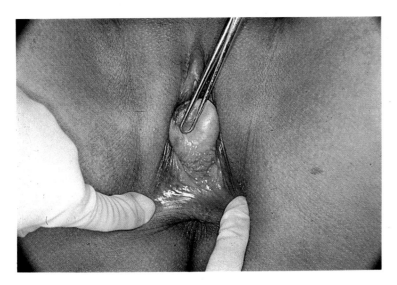

2.45

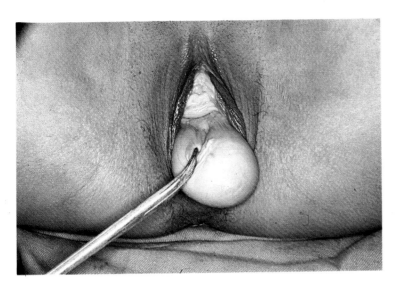

2.46

Benign tumours

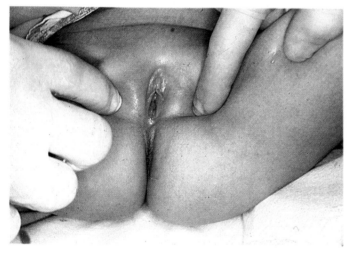

2.47

Figs 2.47 & 2.48 Vaginal Polyp. This is a rare tumour which may be seen in infants (Fig. 2.47) or in adults (Fig. 2.48). The origin from the vaginal mucosa has to be demonstrated to differeniate it from the much more common urethral caruncles, cervical and uterine polypi.

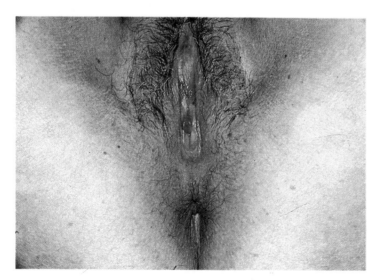

2.48

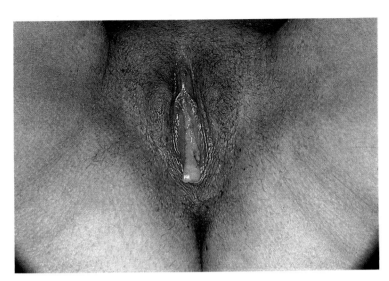

2.49

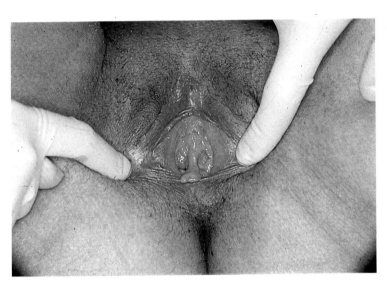

2.50

Figs 2.49 & 2.50 Vaginal Papilloma. True vaginal papillomata are rare tumours. Unlike Bilharzial papillomata they are always solitary. They usually arise in the lower part of the vagina, have a long pedicle and as in Figs 2.49 and 2.50 may protrude from the vaginal introitus.

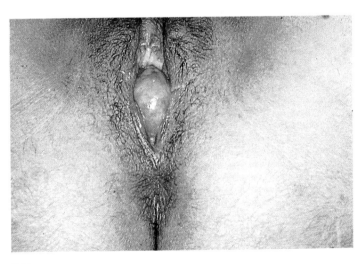

2.51

Fig. 2.51 Fibroma. Fibroma of the vagina is a very rare tumour. It may be pedunculated and appear at the introitus. Clinically it is a firm benign noninfiltrating growth. The true nature of the tumour can only be revealed by histopathological examination.

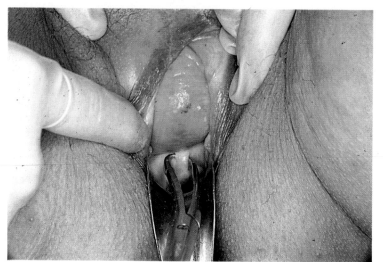

2.52

Fig. 2.52 Fibroma of the Vesicovaginal Septum.
This rare tumour could be mistaken for cystocele
or for a cyst of the anterior vaginal wall. On
palpation the tumour was found to be of firm
consistency. The patient presented with marked
urinary symptoms.

Malignant tumours

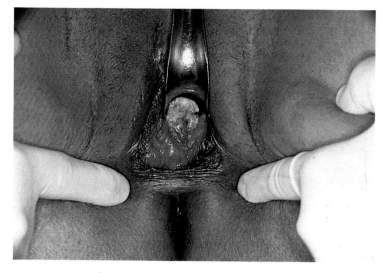

2.53

Figs 2.53–2.55 Carcinoma of the Vagina.
Primary carcinoma of the vagina is rare. Therefore the clinical teaching is that if carcinoma is
also present in the cervix or in the vulva the
lesion in the vagina should, as a rule, be considered secondary.

Figs 2.53–2.55 illustrate the 3 clinical types of
primary carcinoma of the vagina. In Fig. 2.53 the
lesion is of the indurated nodular type. There is
no ulceration or fungation but the growth shows
an infected nodular surface and elevated inverted
edges. There was marked induration and infiltration of the surrounding tissues. Fig. 2.54 shows
an endophytic (ulcerative) lesion which readily
bleeds on touch, also with everted edges and
marked infiltration of the vaginal mucosa. Fig.
2.55 shows an exophytic (fungating) caracinoma.
Although in this case the tumour reaches down

almost to the vulva, the bulk of the lesion is in the vagina which leaves no doubt as to its primary vaginal origin.

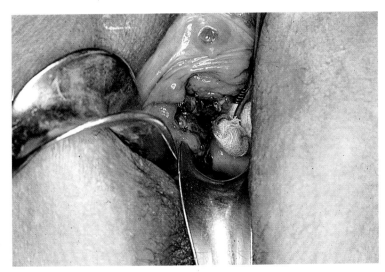

2.54

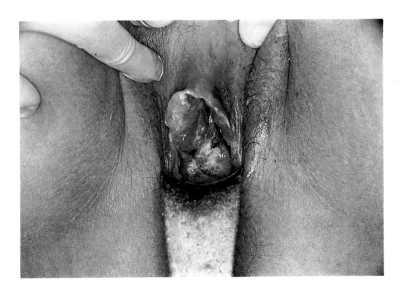

2.55

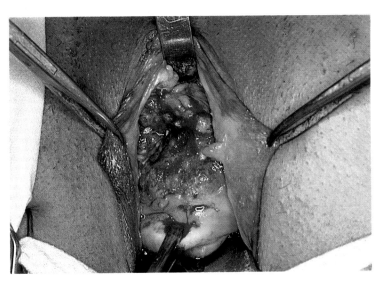

2.56

Fig. 2.56 Bilharzial Carcinoma of the Vagina.
There is evidence that Bilharziasis of the vagina may be precancerous. In this case biopsy showed Bilharzia ova in a well differentiated squamous cell carcinoma. Bilharzial carcinoma of the vagina is often, as in the case shown here, of the indurated nodular type with much less bleeding and friability than non-Bilharzial carcinoma.

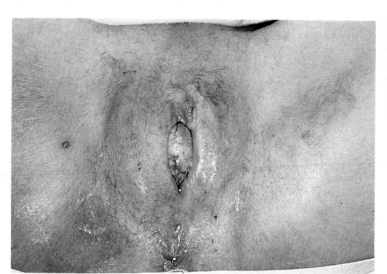

2.57

Figs 2.57 & 2.58 Fibrosaracoma of the Vagina. A rapidly growing tumour arising from the anterior vaginal wall and protruding from the vaginal introitus. Malignancy was suspected because of the old age of the patient, the short history and the ulcerating and infiltrating nature of the tumour. Biopsy showed it to be a fibrosarcoma.

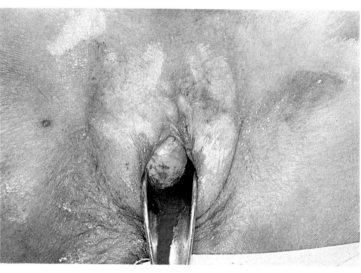

2.58

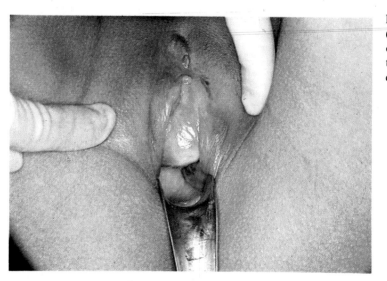

2.59

Fig. 2.59 Choriocarcinoma of the Vagina (Metastatic). The patient had uterine chorio-carcinoma. A single metastatic nodule is seen in the posterolateral wall of the vagina. Note the dark purple colour of the tumour.

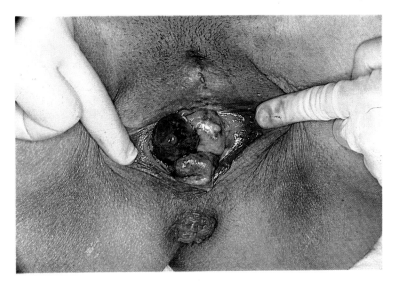

2.60

Fig. 2.60 Malignant Melanoma of the Vagina.
This very rare tumour usually, as in this case, occurs in the lower third of the vagina. The dark brown, almost black, colour of the tumour suggested the correct diagnosis which was confirmed by biopsy.

3. Genital Prolapse

An important step in every gynaecological examination is to ask the patient to bear down strongly, strain or cough while examining the external genitals with the labia separated. This step, which should never be omitted, is essential for the diagnosis of the presence, the type and the degree of genital prolapse.

In examining a case of prolapse, the gynaecologist should look for:

1. The type of prolapse, meaning which parts of the genital tract are involved. There may be prolapse of the anterior vaginal wall, almost always associated with urethrocele and/or cystocele, prolapse of the uterus, prolapse of the posterior vaginal wall with or without rectocele or any combination of these types may be present.

2. The degree of uterine prolapse should be determined with the patient straining maximally. Depending on the level of the uterus, uterine prolapse is classified into three degrees.

3. The presence of associated complications such as perineal or cervical laceration, abnormal pigmentation, vaginitis, cervicitis, ulceration of the vagina, the cervix or rarely even the vulva and erosion, polypi or rarely carcinoma of the cervix.

4. In all cases retroversion of the uterus, supravaginal elongation of the cervix and enterocele (hernia of the Douglas pouch) should be carefully looked for since successful surgical repair entails that if present they should be corrected.

5. The presence of a surgical scar, indicating that the case is one of recurrent prolapse, should also not be missed.

Types of prolapse–
Degrees of uterine
prolapse

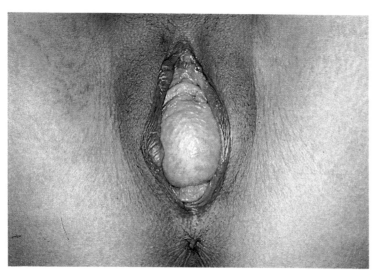

3.1

Fig. 3.1 Cystocele. The anterior vaginal wall protrudes through the vulva. Because of the intimate relation of the bladder to the anterior vaginal wall the rule is that, except in recurrent cases, when the latter prolapses the former always descends in relation to it.

In the case shown there is no uterine descent and the posterior vaginal wall is in its normal position. Note that the prolapsed anterior vaginal wall is stretched and has lost its characteristic transverse folds.

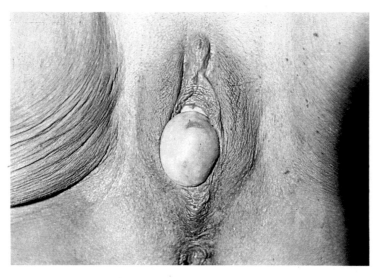

3.2

Figs 3.2 & 3.3 Prolapse of the Posterior Vaginal Wall. Because of the loose cellular tissue of the rectovaginal septum, the rectal wall may or may not follow the descent of the posterior vaginal wall. This can only be determined by rectal examination. In the case shown in Fig. 3.2 there was no rectocele, while in the case shown in Fig. 3.3 the rectum was closely related to the prolapsed posterior vaginal wall (rectocele). In both cases there was almost no uterine descent. Note the absence of rugae in the stretched prolapsed vaginal wall.

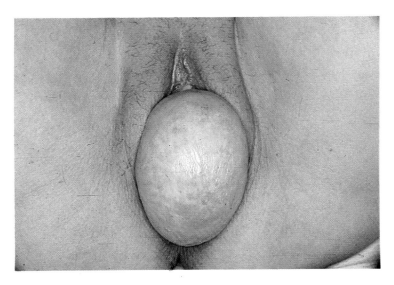

3.3.

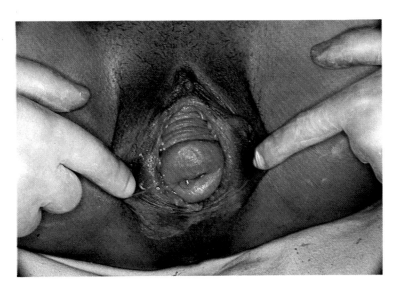

Fig. 3.4 First Degree Uterine Prolapse. On maximal straining the cervix descends below its normal position (the ischial spine plane) but does not actually protrude outside the vulva. There is no prolapse of either vaginal wall. Note the presence of the transverse folds in the vaginal wall.

3.4

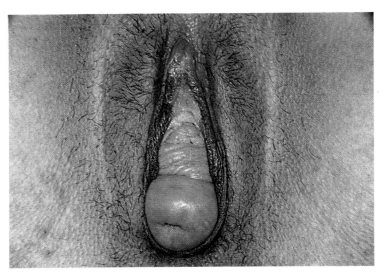

Fig. 3.5 First Degree Uterine Prolapse. Slight Cystocele. On maximal straining the cervix descends down to but not outside the vulva. There is slight descent of the anterior vaginal wall which retains its folds.

3.5

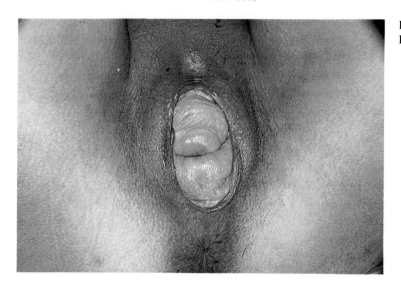

Fig. 3.6 First Degree Uterine Prolapse. Slight Prolapse of Posterior Vaginal Wall.

3.6

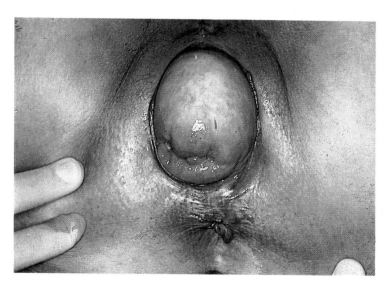

Fig. 3.7 Second Degree Uterine Prolapse. Slight Cystocele. On straining the cervix protrudes outside the vulva but the bulk of the uterus is still inside. There is slight descent of the anterior but not the posterior vaginal wall.

3.7

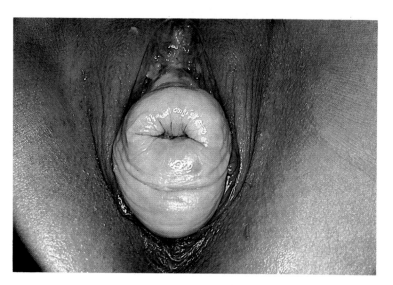

Fig. 3.8 Second Degree Uterine Prolapse. Slight Prolapse of Posterior Vaginal Wall. On straining the cervix and part of posterior vaginal wall descend below the level of the vulva. In this case rectal examination showed that the rectum was in normal position (no rectocele).

3.8

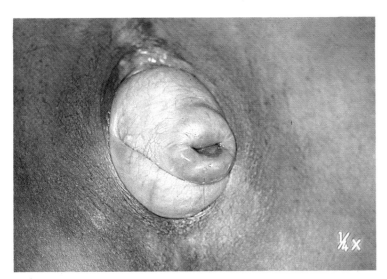

Figs 3.9 & 3.10 Second Degree Uterine Prolapse. Cystorectocele. In these two cases the cervix and part of the uterine body, as well as the anterior and posterior vaginal walls, protruded outside the vulva on straining. In both cases rectal examination showed that rectocele was present.

3.9

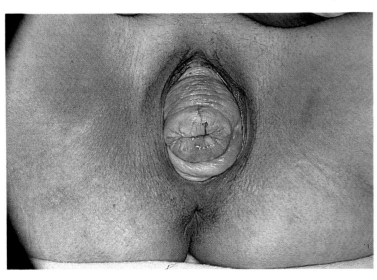

3.10

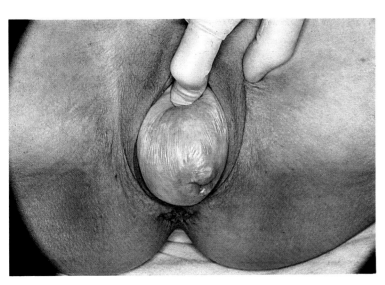

Figs 3.11–3.15 Clinical Tests to Differentiate between Second and Third Degrees of Uterine Prolapse. One finger (Fig. 3.11), two fingers (Figs 3.12, 3.13) or preferably the thumb and fingers (Figs 3.14, 3.15) are placed at the level of the vaginal introitus while the patient is requested to bear down as much as she can. In second degree prolapse (Figs 3.11–3.13) the fingers feel the thickness of the uterus which is still inside the vagina.

In third degree prolapse, also called procidentia, (Figs 3.14, 3.15) only the thin vaginal walls are felt, the entire uterus having descended below the level of the examining fingers. Note that in the more marked degrees of uterine prolapse the utrus is almost invariably retroverted (Fig. 3.15).

3.11

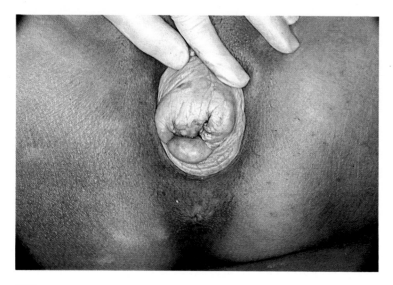

3.12

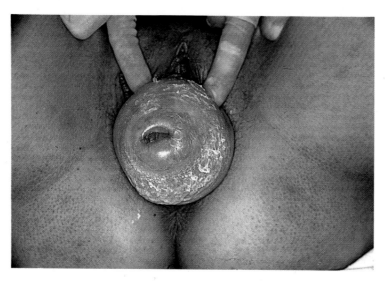

3.13.

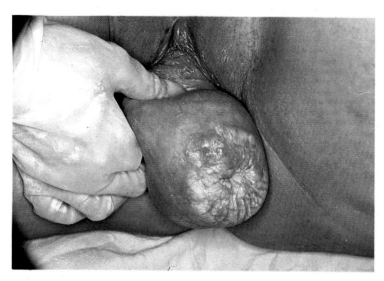

3.14

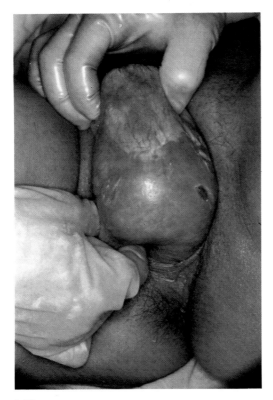

3.15

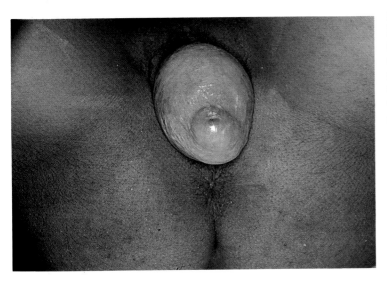

3.16

Figs 3.16 & 3.17 Nulliparous Prolapse. Procidentia. Cystorectocele. Prolapse is uncommon in nulliparous women. It may occur at any age and is essentially due to congenital weakness of the genital supports. Note the small cervix and the small rounded nulliparous external os. The vaginal introitus is much less patulous than in the usual multiparous prolapse.

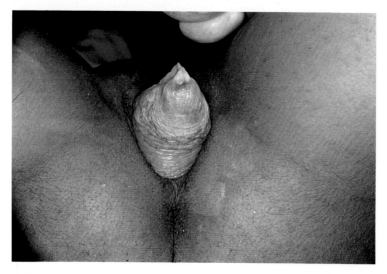

3.17

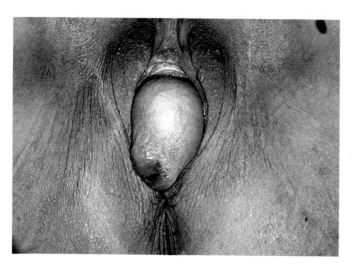

Fig. 3.18 Second Degree Uterine Prolapse and Cystocele in a Nullipara. Note the small cervix and relatively narrow vagina.

3.18

Associated conditions– Complications

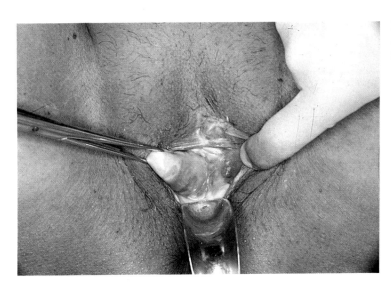

Figs 3.19 & 3.20 Vault Prolapse After Total Abdominal Hysterectomy. The hysterectomy scar is clearly visible in Fig. 3.20. To prevent this complication it is the author's practice always to suspend the vaginal vault to the stumps of the divided parametrium, and round and ovarian (or infundibulopelvic) ligaments.

3.19

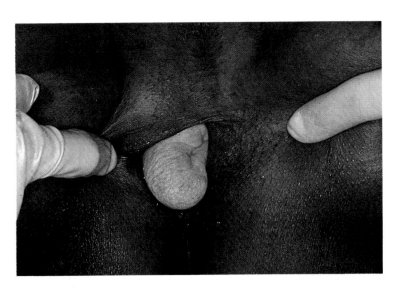

3.20

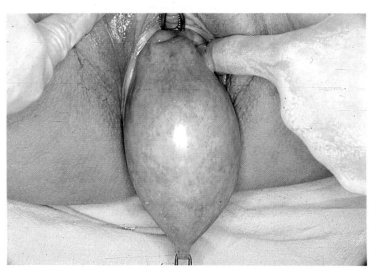

3.21

Fig. 3.21 Enterocele. This may be associated with marked uterine prolapse or may, as in this case, be present with relatively little uterine descent.

The condition is a true hernia of the pouch of Douglas and the bulge starting in the upper posterior wall of the vagina consists of a peritoneal sac frequently containing small bowel.

The mass looks like prolapse of the posterior vagina wall with or without rectocele (see Fig. 3.3) but if the patient is asked to cough with the fingers placed in the posterior fornix or grasping the swelling or with a finger in the rectum a characteristic gurgling sensation can be felt and occasionally seen.

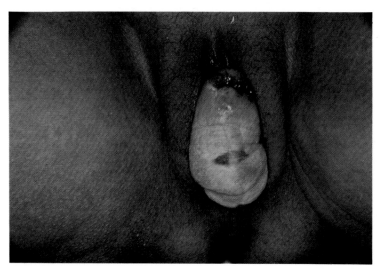

3.22

Figs 3.22 & 3.23 Pigmentation of the Vagina and Cervix. This is not uncommonly seen in cases of prolapse. It may be localized and patchy (Fig. 3.22) or diffuse (Fig. 3.23).

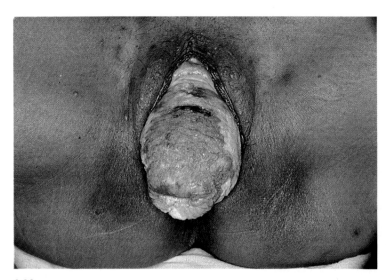

3.23

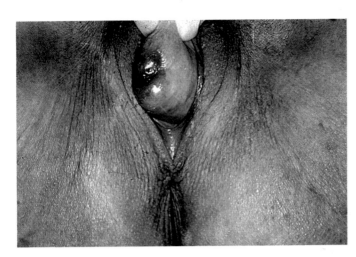

Fig. 3.24 Erosion of the Prolapsed Cervix (see Chapter 5).

3.24

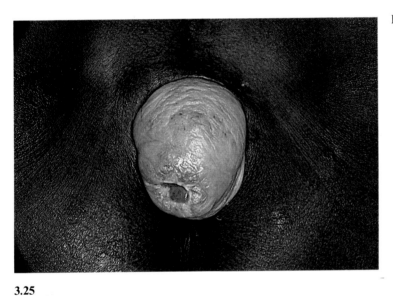

Fig. 3.25 Cervical Polyp with Prolapse.

3.25

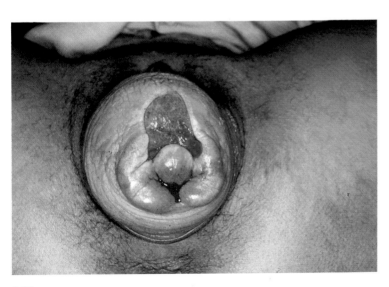

Figs 3.26 & 3.27 Ulceration of the Vagina. This is a common complication of long standing prolapse. It may affect the anterior wall (Fig. 3.26) or the posterior wall (Fig. 3.27) or both. This is due to defective circulation and continuous friction with the underwear.

3.26

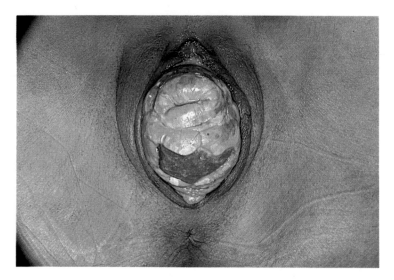

3.27

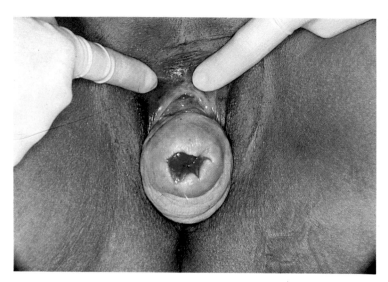

3.28

Figs 3.28 & 3.29 Ulceration of the Cervix. This is also a frequent complication of uterine prolapse. The ulcer in Fig. 3.28 is small, clean and caused little in the way of symptoms. The ulcer in Fig. 3.29 affects almost the entire portio vaginalis of the cervix, it is infected and bled on touch. The patient complained of foul smelling blood-stained discharge. Because of its suspicious appearance biopsy was made and, as in most similar ulcers with prolapse, showed no evidence of malignancy.

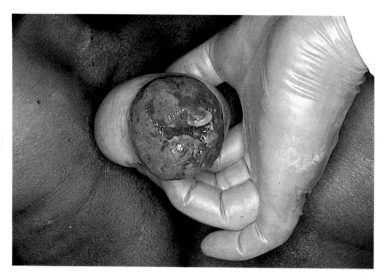

3.29

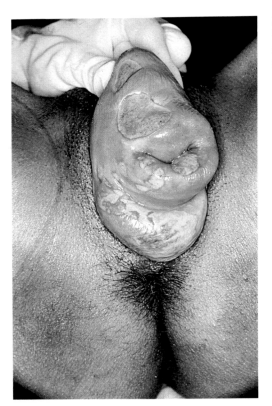

Figs 3.30 & 3.31 Extensive Ulceration of the Vagina and Cervix. Being of similar aetiology, ulcers of the vagina and cervix are often present together in untreated prolapse.

3.30

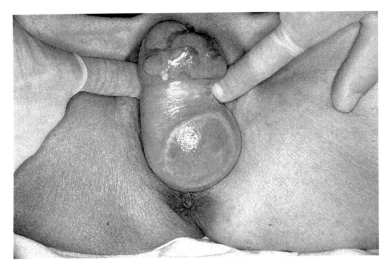

3.31

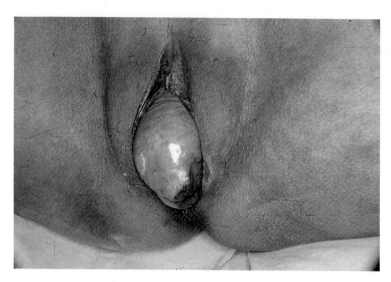

Figs 3.32 & 3.33 Ulceration of the Vulva. This is a very unusual complication of prolapse. In this case prolonged friction caused ulceration of the cervix, the left lateral vaginal wall and the adjacent part of the left labium majus.

3.32

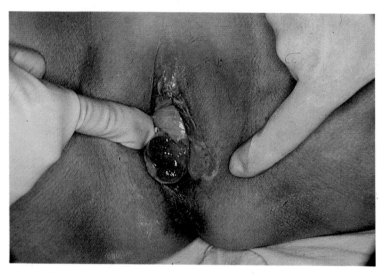

3.33

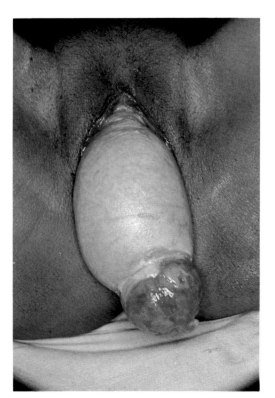

3.34

Figs 3.34 & 3.35 Elongation and Hypertrophy of the Cervix. This is not uncommonly present in cases of second degree (Fig. 3.34) and third degree (Fig. 3.35) uterine prolapse. It is usually more marked in the supravaginal cervix which may be 10 centimetres or more in length, but may also affect the vaginal portion when it is ulcerated and chronically infected (Fig. 3.35).

It is the author's opinion that supravaginal elongation of the cervix with prolapse is not due to stretching but to actual hypertrophy and thickening of the tissues as a result of prolonged lymphatic and venous stasis, congestion and oedema. It is thus similar to the marked thickening of the vaginal walls, especially the anterior, which is also often present (Fig. 3.35).

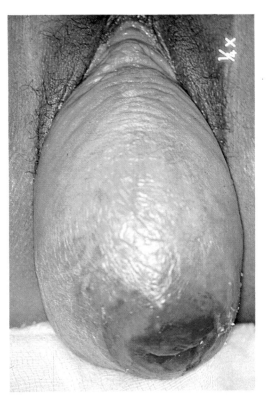

3.35

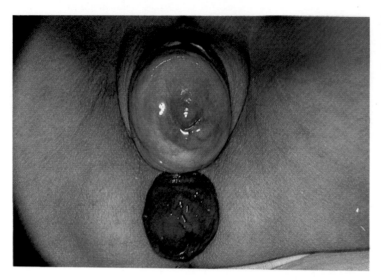

Figs 3.36 & 3.37 Prolapse of the Rectum. Cystorectocele. Second Degree Uterine Prolapse. This association is not common. Most cases are elderly frail women with marked weakness of the pelvic floor.

3.36

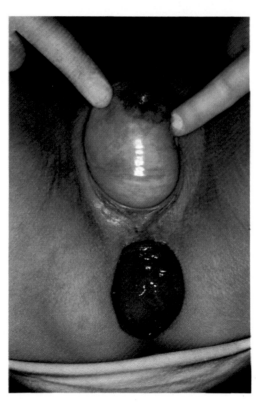

3.37

Recurrent prolapse

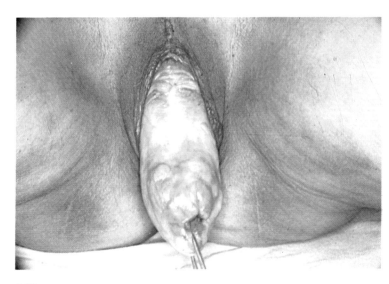

Fig. 3.38 Recurrent Second Degree Uterine Prolapse and Cystorectocele. Note the marked elongation of the supravaginal cervix. The scar of the previous repair operation is clearly seen.

3.38

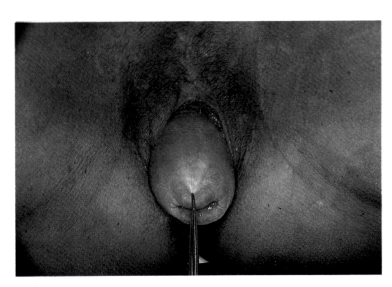

Fig. 3.39 Marked Elongation and Hypertrophy of the Cervix following classical repair of prolapse. This interesting clinical entity may occur if amputation of the cervix in the original repair operation is indicated but not performed. In the case shown the repair was successful in that the uterus and vaginal walls are in normal position but the now much elongated cervix protrudes outside the vulva. Strictly speaking this should not be classified as recurrent prolapse.

3.39

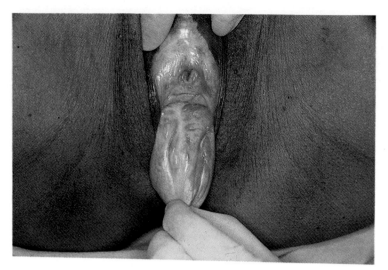

3.40

Figs 3.40 & 3.41 Vault Prolapse Following Vaginal Hysterectomy. This 50-year-old patient had had vaginal hysterectomy and repair for genital prolapse 2 years previously. The vaginal vault is everted together with the whole anterior and posterior vaginal walls, but there is no cystocele (catheter showed bladder in normal position), rectocele or enterocele. The scars of the previous surgery are seen in both vaginal walls.

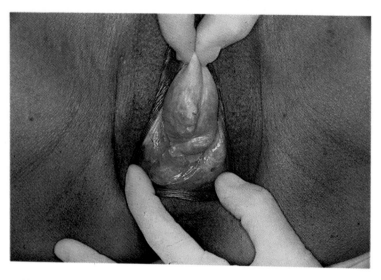

3.41

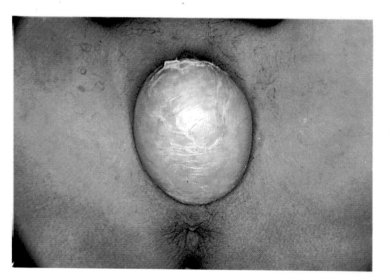

3.42

Fig. 3.42 Vault Prolapse, Rectocele and Enterocele Following Vaginal Hysterectomy. Another case of postmenopausal prolapse recurrent after vaginal hysterectomy. Rectal examination showed that the rectum was closely related to the prolapsed posterior vaginal wall. The mass had an expansile impulse on coughing with distinct gurgling sensation diagnostic of enterocele.

4. Perineal Tears– Rectovaginal Fistula– Genitourinary Fistulas

Perineal tears usually result from birth trauma and may be incomplete or complete. In the latter the anal sphincter is torn and the tear may involve the anal canal and sometimes even the rectum.

Low rectovaginal fistulas are usually the result of incomplete healing or inadequate repair of a complete perineal tear. Rectal fistulas opening higher up in the vagina are more commonly due to surgical or irradiation trauma but may complicate inflammatory conditions, such as an abscess opening both ways, or may rarely be caused by malignant disease of the rectum or the vagina. The most important symptom of rectovaginal fistulas is incontinence of stools..

The most important symptom of genitourinary fistulas is incontinence of urine. The incontinence in cases of fistula is sometimes called 'true' incontinence meaning that the urine passes into and from the vagina. In all other types of incontinence such as sphincteric (stress) incontinence, urgency incontinence and retention with overflow the urine escapes involuntarily from the urethral opening. This is an important diagnostic point which can be determined by history taking and by examination.

Genitourinary fistulas may involve the vagina, the cervix or even the body of the uterus. The communication may be with the urethra, the bladder or the ureter. In urethral fistulas below the bladder neck, the patient is usually continent and may only complain of abnormal urinary stream during micturition as the urine passes into the vagina. In bladder fistulas, there is usually complete urinary incontinence except when the fistula is vary small and valvular when some urine may be retained in the bladder or when the fistula is situated above the level of the uterine isthmus when menouria (Youssef's syndrome)[4] will occur. In ureteric fistulas there is true incontinence with the urine from the injured ureter dribbling into the vagina, but the incontinence is usually partial as the bladder fills from the intact ureter and the patient has normal acts of micturition. Thus careful anamnesis can belp to determine the site of the fistula even before the patient is examined.

In all cases of genital fistula the examiner should, by inspection and palpation, determine the site, size, shape and mobility of the fistula, the presence of more than one fistular opening, the presence of other associated injuries such as perineal or cervical laceration and the presence of such complications as urinary calculus and inflammation of the genital and/or urinary tract.

Other techniques used in the investigation of urinary fistulas include the injection of methylene blue solution into the bladder to help determine the site of fistula, cystoscopy and intravenous pyelography.

Perineal tears

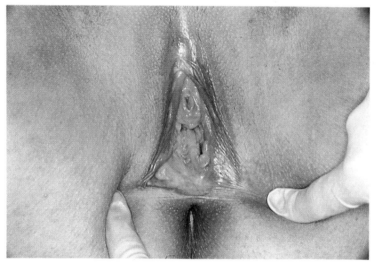

Fig. 4.1 Incomplete Perineal Tear (First Degree). The scar involves the anterior part of the perineal body.

4.1

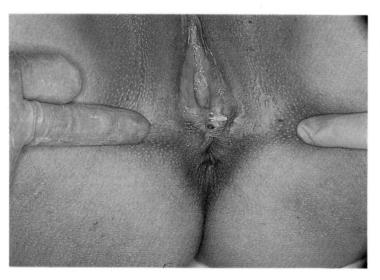

Fig. 4.2 Incomplete Perineal Tear (Second Degree). The tear extends to but does not include the external sphincter of the anus. The presence and extent of perineal tears can only be diagnosed with the labia separated.

4.2

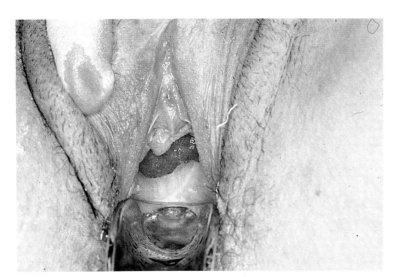

4.21

Figs 4.21–4.23 Large Vesicovaginal Fistula.
When the fistula is large, the bladder mucosa may be visible through the abnormal opening. It is recognized by its bright red colour. The position and extent of the fistula can be demonstrated by the introduction of a metal catheter.

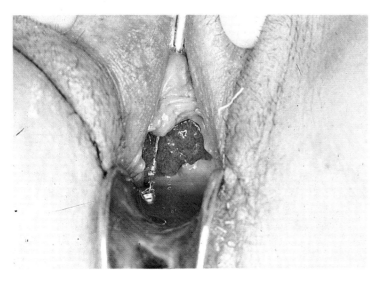

4.22

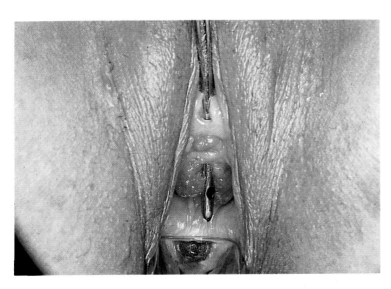

4.23

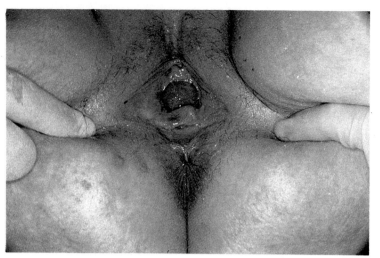

4.24

Figs 4.24–4.26, 4.27 Huge Vesicovaginal Fistula.
When most of the anterior vaginal wall and
bladder base slough away, and this is almost
always the result of obstructed labour, the re-
maining bladder mucosa may protrude into the
vagina, as in the two cases shown, simulating a
polyp or a tumour. The diagnosis is made from
the history, the complete urinary incontinence
and the bright red colour of the bladder mucosa.
It is confirmed by the passage of a catheter into
the urethra (Fig. 4.26) or what remains of it (Fig.
4.27).

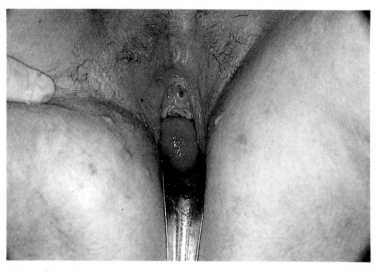

4.25

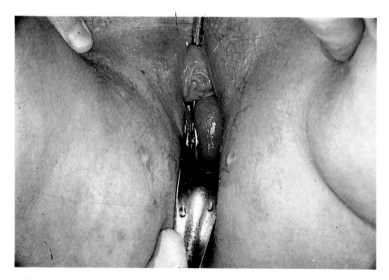

4.26

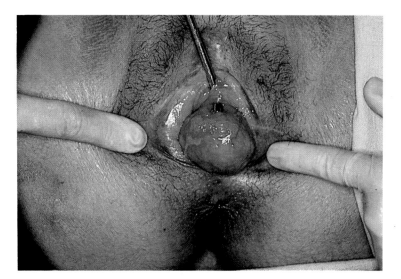

4.27

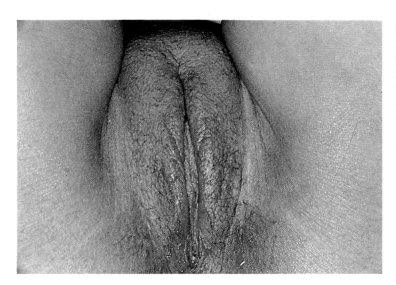

4.28

Figs 4.28 & 4.29 Vesicovaginal Fistula. Vulvitis.
Vulvitis is a common complication of untreated
cases of genitourinary fistulas and is due to the
irritation caused by the continuous dribbling of
urine. The vulva may be red and oedematous
(Fig. 4.28) and there may be widespread furunculosis (Fig. 4.29) and ulceration. The skin of the
perineum, perianal region and buttocks may
share in the inflammatory process.

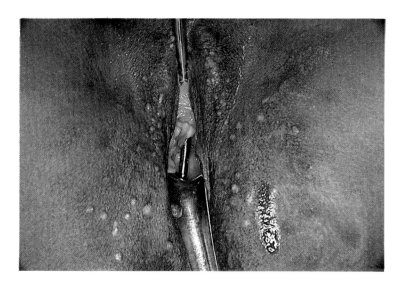

4.29

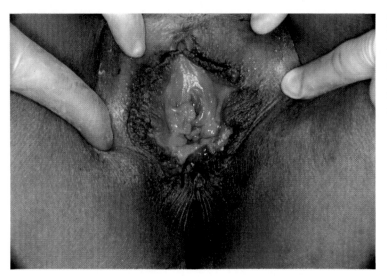

4.30

Fig. 4.30 Vesicovaginal Fistula. Complete Perineal Tear. In all cases of geniturinary fistulas, especially those following delivery, careful search should be made for other genital injuries which may have resulted from the same mismanagement. In the case shown the not uncommon association of vesicovaginal fistula and complete perineal tear is demonstrated.

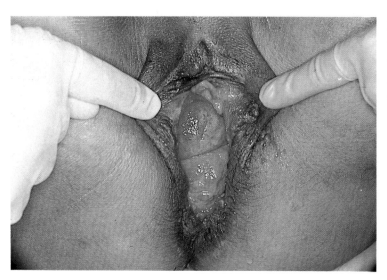

4.31

Figs 4.31 & 4.32 Large Vesicovaginal Fistula. Complete Perineal Tear. A very large vesicovaginal fistula with prolapse of the bladder mucosa as well as a third degree perineal tear after difficult labour. The patient was under treatment for vulvitis but a few small boils are still seen near the left labium majus.

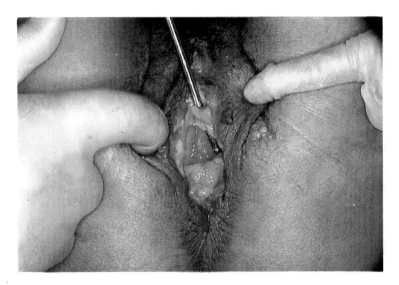

4.32

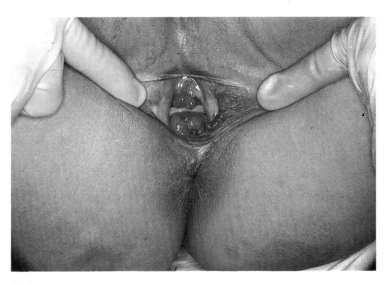

4.33

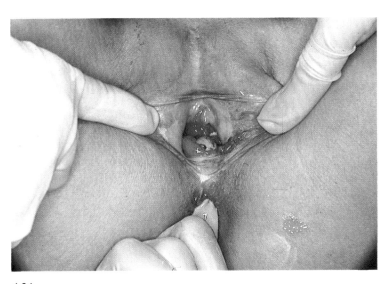

4.34

Figs 4.33 & 4.34 Large Vesicovaginal Fistula. Rectovaginal Fistula. In this 20-year-old unipara, a prolonged obstructed labour was terminated by a difficult forceps delivery in a small provincial hospital. There is a large vesicovaginal fistula with prolapse of the bladder mucosa and a large rectovaginal fistula which easily admits a finger.

The bladder fistula was probably the result of sloughing and necrosis and the rectal fistula of direct injury by the forceps. Note the similar bright red colour of the bladder and rectal mucosa which is quite different from the pale pink colour of the vaginal mucosa.

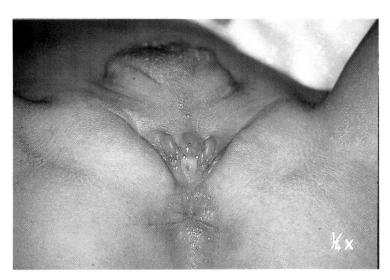

4.35

Fig. 4.35 Ectopia Vesica. Congenital absence of the anterior wall of the bladder and urethra, the symphysial junction and the lower part of the anterior abdominal wall. The mucous membrane seen is that of the posterior bladder wall. There was complete urinary incontinence. Note scar of previous unsuccessful attempt at surgical repair.

5. Diseases of the Cervix Uteri

Exposure of the cervix with a speculum is a must in every gynaecological examination. A self retaining bivalvular speculum is most suitable for this purpose, but occasionally other types of specula and retractors may be needed.

It is well known that certain very common lesions of the cervix, such as 'erosions' and polypi are often much better seen than felt. For this reason, and because, in my experience, students usually find difficulty in their differential diagnosis, these two entities are herein amply illustrated and described in detail.

'Erosion' of the cervix must be differentiated from the true ulcer of the cervix; in the former the squamous epithelium outside the external os is replaced by columnar epithelium while in the latter there is actual loss of the epithelial surface. Aetiologically, erosions are classified as being of congenital, hormonal or inflammatory origin. Clinically, they are classified into the simple flat, the papillary and the follicular types.

By far the commonest type of cervical polyp is the mucous polyp. This may be single or multiple and is usually small. If it grows much in size it may exhibit different structural patterns. Thus adenomatous (prepondrance of glandular tissue), fibroadenomatous (prepondrance of fibrous tissue) and cystic (obstruction of glandular ducts) types are recognized. The differential diagnosis between the large cervical polyp and the not uncommon uterine fibroid polyp protruding through the cervix is discussed in this chapter and in Chapter 6. An important point in differentiating between cervical and corporeal polypi can only be determined by palpation. In the former the pedicle is found to arise from the cervical canal; in the latter it can be traced to the inside of the uterine cavity.

In the author's opinion the 'unhealthy' cervix plays an important role in the aetiology of female infertility. Abnormalities which may seem slight or insignificant are sometimes the only cause for the failure to conceive. The dilatation of a narrow cervical canal, the clearing of hostile cervical mucus, the treatment of cervical infection or the cauterisation of an erosion may be followed by successful pregnancy.

Benign tumours of the cervix are uncommon. Carcinoma of the cervix, on the other hand is the commonest of all malignant diseases of the female genital tract. The early detection of carcinoma of the cervix depends not only on very careful inspection of the organ but also on the use of such techniques as colposcopy, cytology, endocervical curettage and biopsy.

Congenital–Mechanical–Inflammation

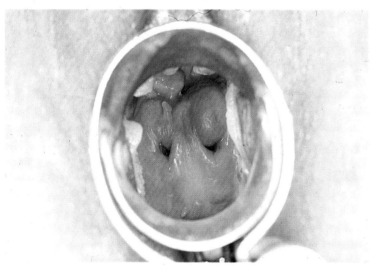

Fig. 5.1 Duplication of the Cervix. Uterus Bicornis Bicollis. This patient had duplication of the cervix but not the vagina. The abnormality may be missed if careful palpation and speculum examination are not carried out.

5.1

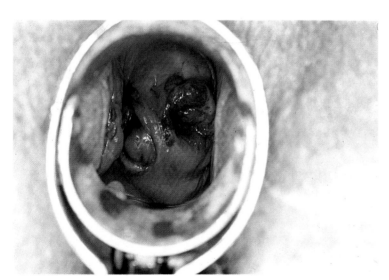

Fig. 5.2 Duplication of the Cervix. Uterus Bicornis Bicollis. This patient had had a recent mid-trimester abortion, hence the dialated left cervix and the blood stained oedematous tissues

It has been shown by the author that repeated abortion in cases of uterine duplication is much more often due to associated congenital incompetence of the isthmus than to the duplication itself. Such cases should be treated by circlage rather than by a unification operation.[5]

5.2

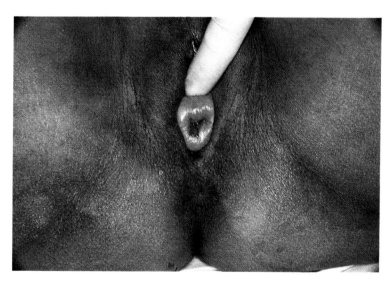

5.3

Fig. 5.3 Congenital Elongation of the Cervix.
This patient was a nullipara with no genital prolapse. In this rare condition the portio vaginalis
of the cervix is long and, unlike in prolapse, it
tapers toward the external os. The vaginal for-
nices are deep. Straining causes no abnormal
descent. In this case the elongated cervix reached
down to the level of the vulva. A small polyp
happens to be present at the external os.

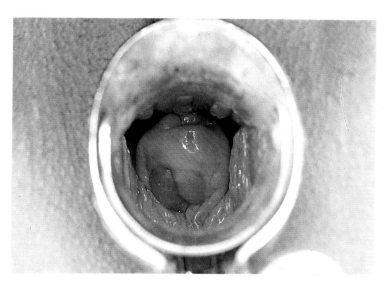

5.4

Figs 5.4 & 5.5 Posterior Cervicovaginal Fistula.
A not very uncommon complication of the
Shirodkar operation. Through a tear in the
posterior wall of the cervix the cervical canal
communicates with the vagina. This patient
complained of secondary infertility.

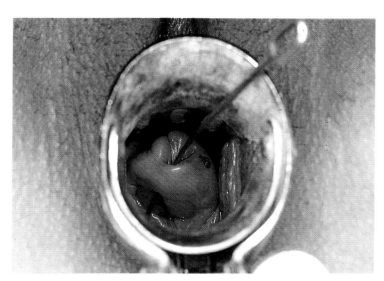

5.5

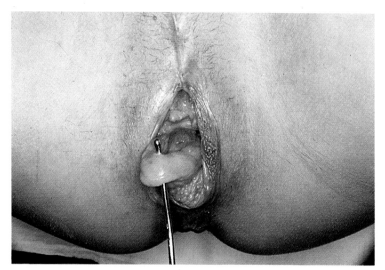

5.6

Fig. 5.6 Anterior Cervicovaginal Fistula. This also occurred after a Shirodkar operation. The vaginal portion of the cervix is abnormally long and the tear here is in the anterior lip.

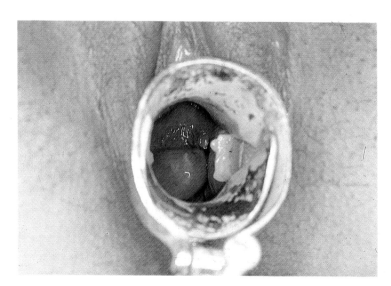

5.7

Fig. 5.7 Bilateral Cervical Tear. Cervical tears are almost always a complication of labour. They are often, as in this case, associated with chronic inflammation of the cervix.

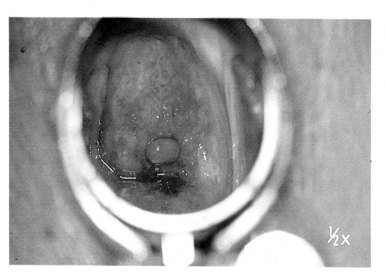

5.8

Fig. 5.8 Right Cervical Tear. Postpartum cervical tears are sometimes unilateral. In this case there is an extensive right sided laceration associated with chronic infection and hypertrophy of the anterior lip of the cervix.

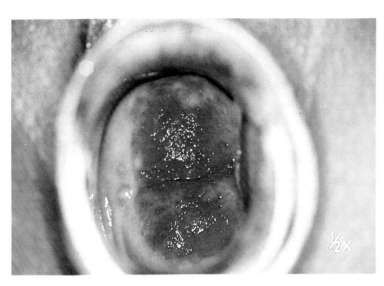

Fig. 5.9 Ectropion. In cases of deep bilateral cervical tears hypertrophy and fibrosis of the cervical lips may occur. The cervical lips are everted exposing a large area of the endocervical mucosa which has an intense red colour. This should be differentiated from cervical erosion (see p. 125) in which the columnar epithelium covered red area is present outside the external os.

5.9

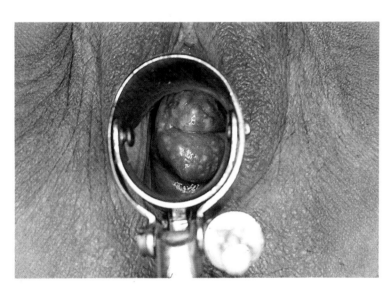

Fig. 5.10 Ectropion. In this case a transformation zone is seen inside the cervical canal with the formation of many Nabothian follicles due to obstruction of the cervical glands by growing squamous epithelium. This is similar to the healing process in so called erosions (see p. 128) but here the changes occur inside the exposed cervical canal.

5.10

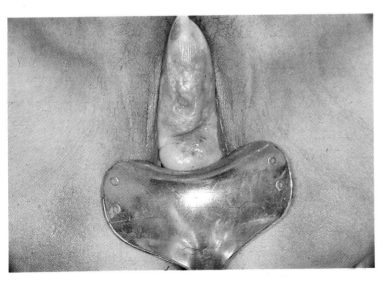

Fig. 5.11 Ectropion. Here there is ectropion of the cervix associated with first degree uterine prolapse.

5.11

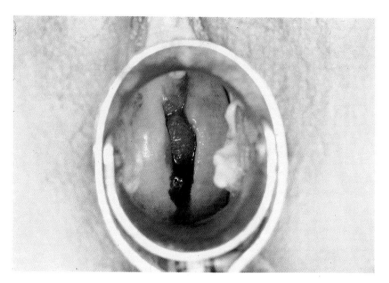

5.12

Fig. 5.12 Ulcer of the Cervix. A true ulcer with loss of the epithelial covering is seen in the anterior lip of the cervix.

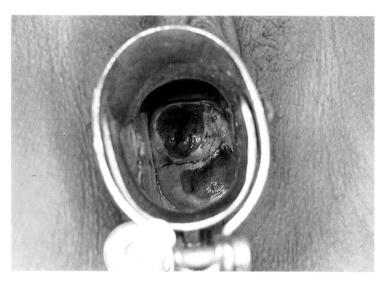

5.13

Fig. 5.13 Ulcers of the Cervix and Vagina. A true ulcer is seen surrounding the external cervical os and another in the posterior vaginal wall. In this patient the ulcers resulted from the use of a Hodge pessary for the correction of retroverted uterus! In the author's opinion, there is no place for pessary treatment in modern gynaecological practice.

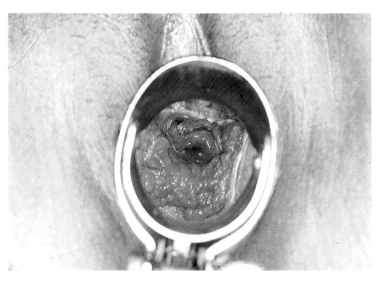

5.14

Figs 5.14 & 5.15 Bilharziasis of the Cervix. In both these cases the lesion presents as multiple small sessile papillomata covered by a rough intact greyish (Fig. 5.14) or pinkish (Fig. 5.15) mucous membrane. In the case shown in Fig. 5.14 the upper vagina is also affected.

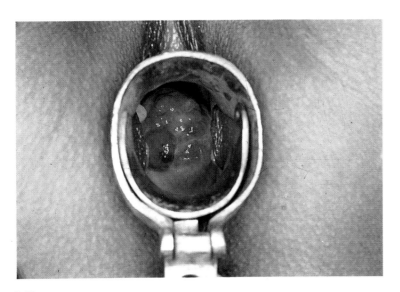

5.15

Cervical erosion

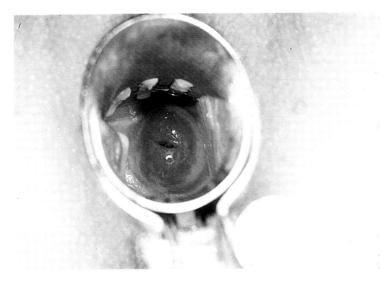

Figs 5.16 & 5.17 Simple Flat Erosion. The term 'erosion' which is used to describe one of the commonest gynaecological conditions, namely a red area in the neighbourhood of the external cervical os, is a misnomer. This term implies loss of tissue at the surface which is now known not to be the case.

The deep red colour is due to the fact that the lesion is covered, not by multilayered squamous epithelium like the normal portio, but by a single layered columnar epithelium through which the capillaries shine.

The term 'erythroplakia' has recently been suggested[6] to replace 'erosion', but the much better known term 'erosion' will be used here.

It is now believed that most erosions are not due to cervicitis but are congenital or predisposed

5.16

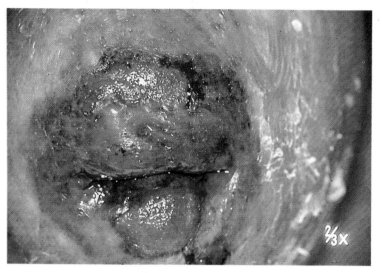

5.17

to by hormonal influences especially those related to pregnancy and labour. Secondary infection, however, commonly occurs.

The erosion may be complete and surround the external os (Figs 5.16, 5.17) or may be patchy. In the two cases shown the erosion is of the simple flat type. The case shown in Fig. 5.16 was an 18-year-old recently married nullipara; the erosion is bright red in colour, covered by clear mucoid discharge, shows no evidence of infection and is probably of congenital origin. In Fig. 5.17 the patient was multiparous and the condition was probably related to pregnancy and labour. Secondary infection was present as evidenced by cervical hypertrophy, tenderness and the presence of mucopurulent discharge which was wiped off before taking the picture.

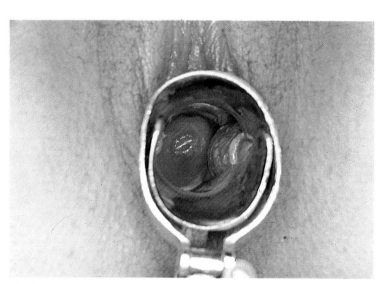

5.18

Figs 5.18–5.20 Papillary Erosion. The basic tendency of columnar epithelium to form rugae and grooves may result in a granular appearance of the erosion and when this process is pronounced the erosion is described as papillary. In these examples, the erosion surrounds the whole external os but sometimes it may be present on one lip only. The papillae may be very small (Fig. 5.18) or fairly large (Fig. 5.19) or the rugae may give the appearance of elevated transverse folds (Fig. 5.20).

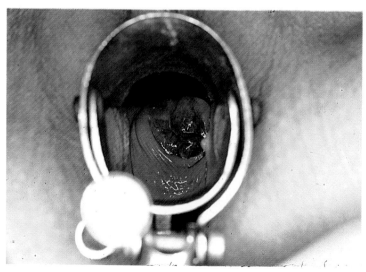

5.19

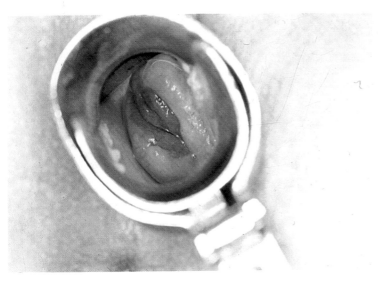

5.20

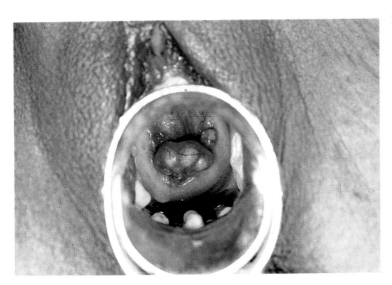

5.21

Fig. 5.21 Follicular (Cystic) Erosion. The continuous interplay between columnar and squamous epithelium as the latter again and again replaces the former in the so-called transformation zone results in the blockage of the ducts of the cervical glands with formation of Nabothian follicles. If this condition is very marked it results in a follicular (cystic) erosion (Fig. 5.20). The small cysts project as tense, shining, yellowish grey rounded bodies of varying size on the cervix.

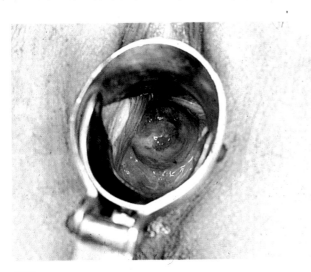

5.22

Fig. 5.22 Cervical Erosion in Pregnancy. Since pregnancy appears to play a role in the pathogenesis of erosion, the latter is a common finding in the cervix during pregnancy. Note the contrast between the bright red colour of the erosion and the dark blue colour of the pregnant cervix.

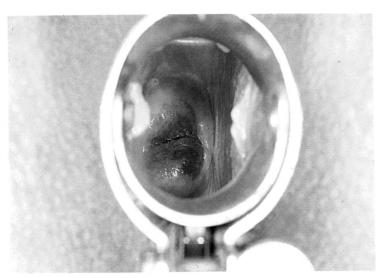

Fig. 5.23 Cervical Erosion in a Pill User.
Papillary erosion surrounding the external os in a woman using oral contraception. Erosions especially of the papillary type are commonly found in pill users.

In pill users the cervix often has a bluish colour not unlike that of the cervix during pregnancy (see Fig. 5.22).

5.23

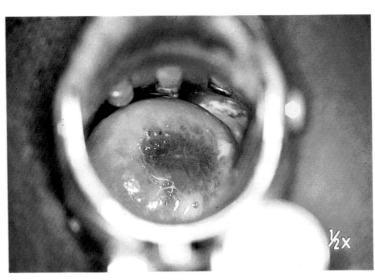

Figs 5.24 & 5.25 Healing Erosion. An erosion, with or without treatment, may be seen in the so-called healing stage. This is actually a transformation zone in which, for the time being, much of the columnar epithelium has been replaced by squamous epithelium. The erosion now is of a much paler colour, is less vascular, has less well defined borders and small Nabothian follicles are often present.

5.24

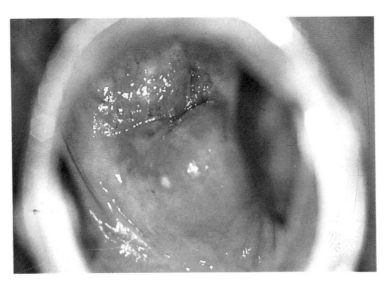

5.25

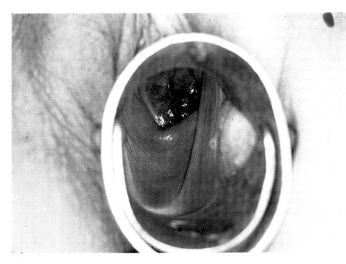

Figs 5.26 & 5.27 Cervical Erosion. Starting Polyp Formation. It is now believed that mucous polypi of the cervix (see p. 130) are the result of focal hyperplasia of the endocervical mucosa. They represent the pronounced tendency of the columnar epithelium in a certain area to become thrown up into projections and folds. In other words a mucous polyp may be regarded as a very localized and very pronounced area of papillary erosion. It is therefore not unusual to find mucous polypi in association with papillary erosion (Figs 5.26 and 5.27).

5.26

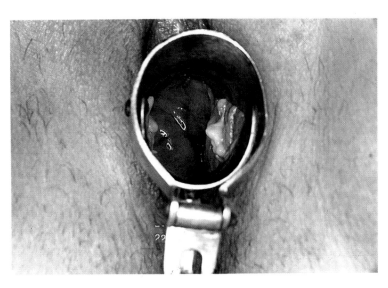

5.27

Cervical polyp

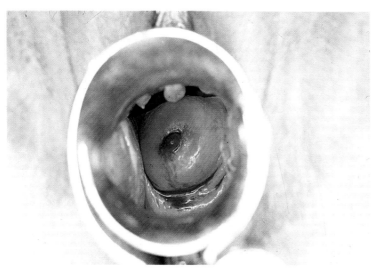

Figs 5.28 & 5.29 Mucous Polyp. A mucous polyp presents as a smooth soft rounded or slightly elongated cherry red structure at the external cervical os. It is usually single, not more than 1 to 1.5 centimetres in length. It usually has a short pedicle but may be sessile.

It most commonly arises inside the cervical canal but may occasionally arise externally from the columnar epithelium of an erosion. If small it can be better seen than felt and may be missed if a speculum is not used. Note the abundant clear mucus and the tendency to bleeding.

5.28

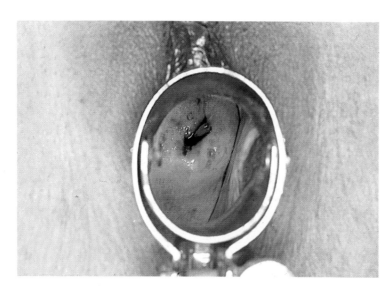

5.29

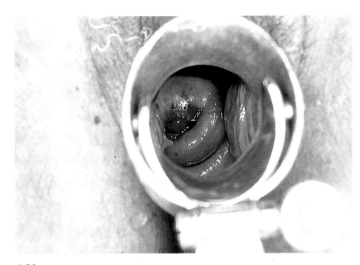

Figs 5.30–5.32 Multiple Mucous Polypi. Not uncommonly two polypi, rarely more, may be seen at the external os. One of them is almost always distinctly larger than the other. Sometimes the difference in size is quite marked (Fig. 5.32), in which case the smaller polyp is always more vascular and its more typical appearance points to the right diagnosis.

5.30

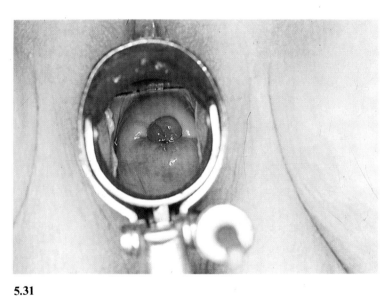

5.31

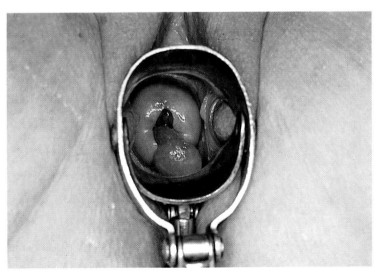

5.32

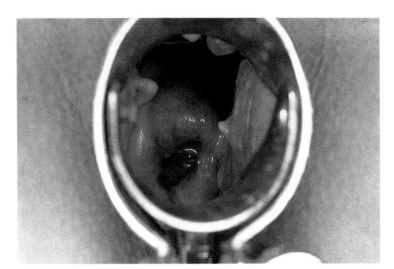

5.33

Fig. 5.33 Mucous Polyp (Adenomatous Type). As mucous polypi become larger in size they may exhibit, microscopically and macroscopically, a variety of structural patterns. When there is preponderance of glandular tissue the polyp more or less retains its typical appearance.

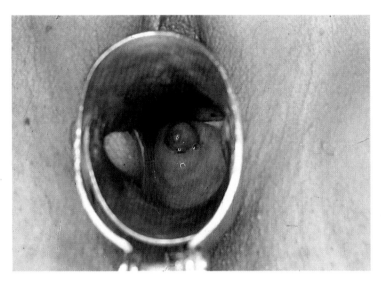

5.34

Figs 5.34–5.36 Mucous Polyp (Cystic Type). Obstruction of the glandular ducts with formation of cystic Nabothian follicles may give the polyp a distinctly cystic appearance. When this process is very marked the polyp may be transformed to what is sometimes called a cyst of the cervix (Fig. 5.36).

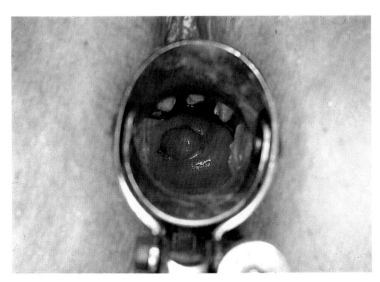

5.35

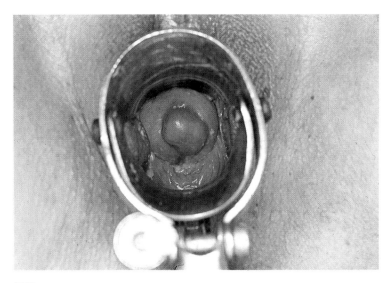

5.36

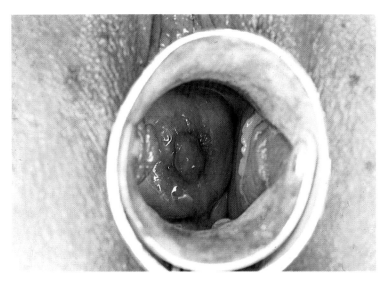

Fig. 5.37 Mucous Polyp (Fibroadenomatous Type). When there is overgrowth of the connective tissue stroma the polyp may be firmer in consistency, less vascular and paler in colour. Sometimes even in such cases vascularity is marked and contact bleeding may still be the chief symptom.

5.37

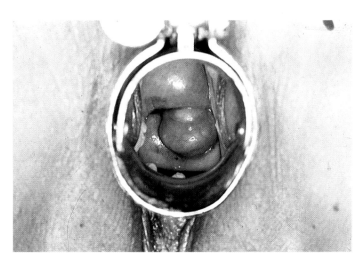

Figs 5.38 & 5.39 Large Mucous Polyp. Large mucous polypi, especially of the fibroadenomatous type, may be very difficult to distinguish clinically from small fibroid polypi (see p. 150), but certain points may help in the differential diagnosis.

Comparing Figs 5.38 & 5.39 with Figs 6.1–6.3 will show that in fibroid polypi the cervical canal is much wider and its external os more circular. The fibroid polyp has a globular shape that is different from the flattened indented appearance of the large mucous polyp which has given rise to the term 'leaf polypi'. The final diagnosis should of course be made by histopathological examination.

5.38

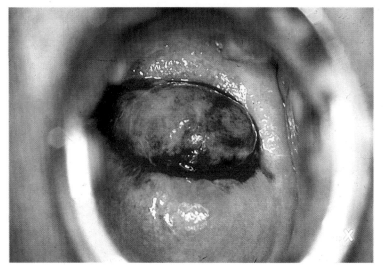

5.39

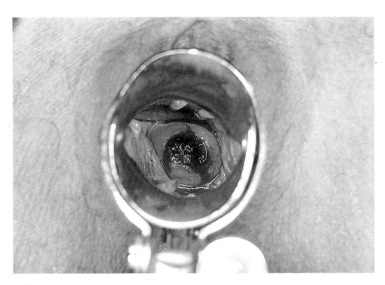

5.40

Figs 5.40 & 5.41 Necrotic Mucous Polyp.
Because of its vascularity a mucous polyp rarely
undergoes sloughing and necrosis. This, however,
may occasionally take place in larger polypi.
Note the dark, almost black colour of the gangrenous polyp.

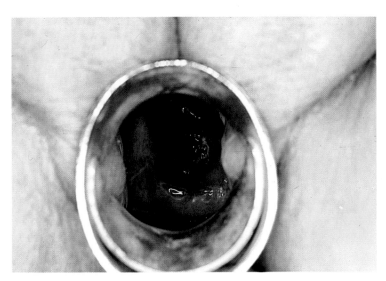

5.41

Benign tumours

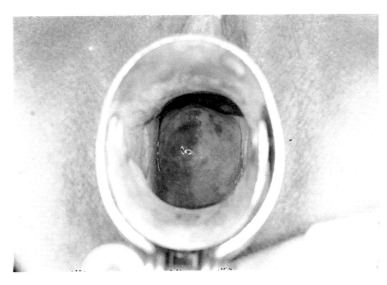

Fig. 5.42 Diffuse Capillary Haemangioma. This is a very rare tumour. Note its dark purplish colour. Microscopic examination showed collections of endothelium-lined blood vessels surrounded by fibrous tissue.

5.42

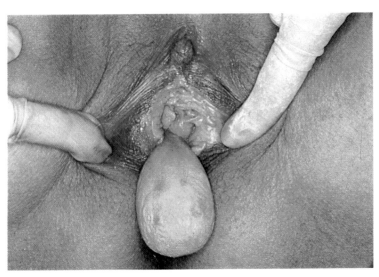

Figs 5.43 & 5.44 Fibroma. Although fibroid (fibromyoma) of the cervix, a tumour which gives rise to no visible physical signs, is by no means uncommon, a pedunculated fibroma arising from the cervix, like the one shown, is exceedingly rare. In this case the patient presented with a mass protruding from the vulva which she thought was genital prolapse. At first sight the mass looked like a large vaginal cyst (see Figs 2.35–2.46), but palpation showed it to be firm in consistency and it was seen to arise from the anterior lip of the cervix. Microscopic examination showed that it was a benign fibroma.

5.43

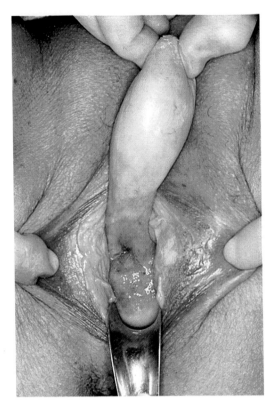

5.44

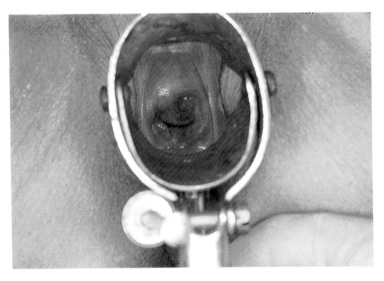

5.45

Figs 5.45–5.48 Suspicious Cervix. In many cases of preinvasive and early invasive carcinoma the cervix shows little in the way of physical signs. In such cases the suspicion of carcinoma and the ultimate diagnosis depend on the use of cytology, colposcopy, curettage and biopsy. But sometimes abnormal appearances in the cervix draw the attention of the wary examiner to the possibility of early malignancy.

In Fig. 5.45 there is a slightly elevated granular lesion at the border of the transformation zone in the anterior lip at about one o'clock. This bled readily on touch and was Schiller's iodine negative. Biopsy showed preinvasive carcinoma.

In Fig. 5.46 a papillary erosion was thought suspicious because of friability and profuse bleeding on examination. Biopsy showed preinvasive carcinoma.

In Fig. 5.47 a somewhat large cervical mucous-like polyp was subjected as usual to histological examination after removal. This showed squamous metaplasia and early invasive carcinoma.

In Fig. 5.48 an elevated granular lesion at the anterior margin of the external os was found to bleed easily on touch. Colposcopy (see p. 144) showed abnormal vascular patterns and an iodine negative area of leukoplakic ground. Biopsy showed early invasive squamous cell carcinoma.

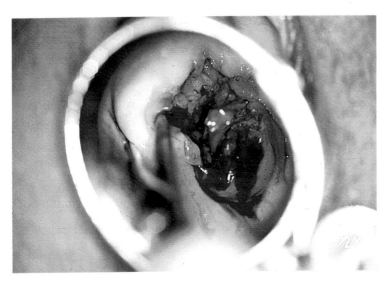

5.46

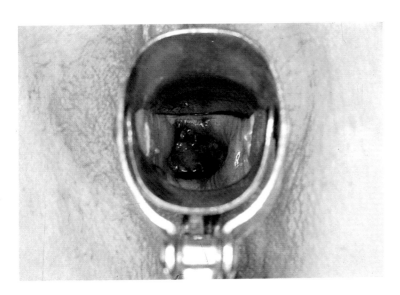

5.47

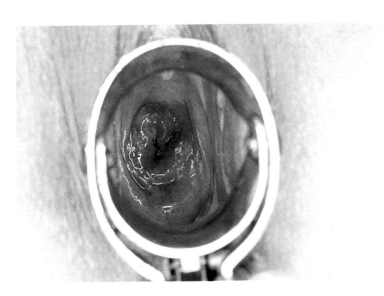

5.48

Carcinoma

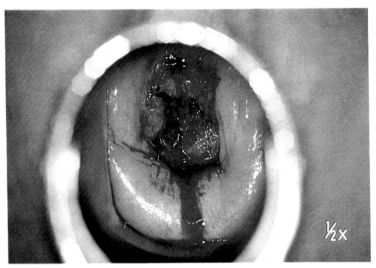

5.49

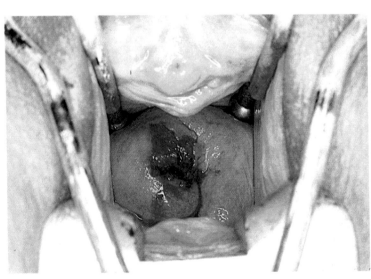

5.50

Figs 5.49–5.52 Stage I Carcinoma. Sometimes the physical signs in the cervix are such as to make the examiner almost certain of the diagnosis of invasive carcinoma although the lesion may still be entirely confined to the cervix. Needless to say, in all cases microscopic examination is mandatory. The carcinoma may originate inside the cervical canal (Fig. 5.49, endocervical) or from a transformation zone at or outside the external os (Figs 5.50–5.52).

In Fig. 5.49 the polypoid growth inside the cervical canal is friable and necrotic and there was considerable bleeding on examination. The lesion, however, was localized to the cervix. The clinical diagnosis of invasive carcinoma was confirmed by microscopic examination.

In Fig. 5.50 there is a true ulcer of the anterior lip of the cervix. The loss of surface epithelium is apparent and distinguishes the lesion from a so called erosion. The base of the ulcer was friable and bled profusely on examination. Biopsy confirmed the clinical diagnosis of invasive carcinoma.

In Fig. 5.51 there is a much deeper excavating ulcer which is strictly confined to the anterior lip. The base of the ulcer is infected, friable and bled readily on touch. Histological examination confirmed the diagnosis of invasive carcinoma.

In Fig. 5.52 unlike the two last cases of ulcerative carcinoma, are seen three nodular growths at the external os. The larger one on the anterior lip showed evidence of breakdown and bleeding on manipulation. There was induration and infiltration of the surrounding tissues but the process was strictly confined to the cervix. The clinical diagnosis of invasive carcinoma was confirmed by biopsy.

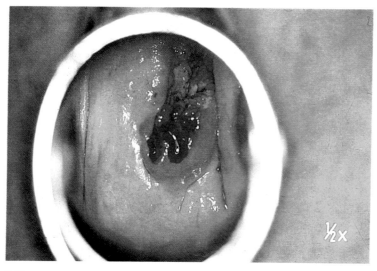

5.51

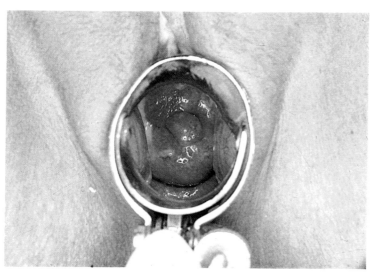

5.52

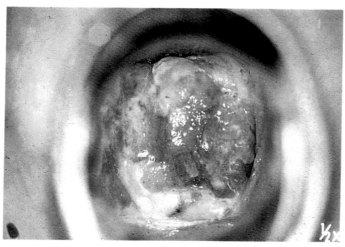

5.53

Figs 5.53–5.65 Advanced Carcinoma. In the case shown in Fig. 5.53 there was parametric infiltration not reaching the pelvic wall (Stage II). The lesions although advanced can still be seen to arise from inside the cervical canal (endo-cervical). The cervix has the characteristic barrel shape of endocervical carcinoma. In cases with more widespread destruction and infiltration it becomes impossible to determine whether the lesion is primarily endocervical or exocervical.

Figs 5.54–5.58 show endophytic (ulcerative) carcinoma. In this condition the lesion forms an excavataing ulcer with irregular shape, granular edges and a friable nodular base that bleeds readily and may be covered by a dirty greyish slough. The process gradually destroys the cervix and infiltrates the parametrium and/or the va-ginal walls.

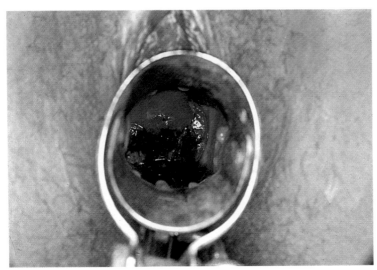

In Fig. 5.54 the ulcerative process has eaten up the posterior lip of the cervix. In Fig. 5.55 the ulcer has destroyed most of the cervix and infiltrated the posterolateral vaginal wall. In Fig. 5.56 the ulcer involves the entire circumference of the cervix. In Fig. 5.57 the ulcerative lesion has infiltrated the entire cervix and spread to both anterior and posterior vaginal walls.

Fig. 5.58 shows bilharzial carcinoma of the cervix. The ulcerative lesion in the anterior lip has infiltrated the anterior vaginal wall. Note that even in advanced cases of bilharzial carcinoma there is much less bleeding and friability than in nonbilharzial lesions. The lesion in this case shows great similarity to the bilharzial vaginal carcinoma shown in Fig. 2.56.

5.54

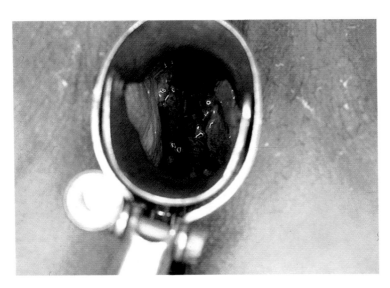

5.55

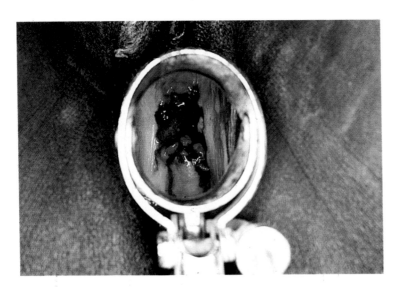

5.56

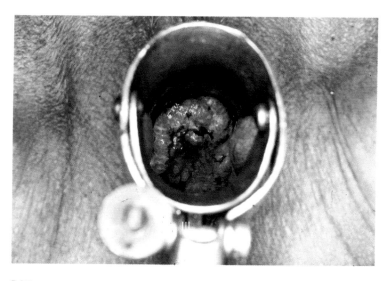

5.57

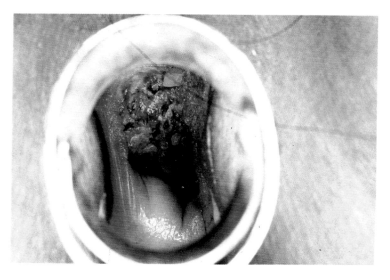

5.58

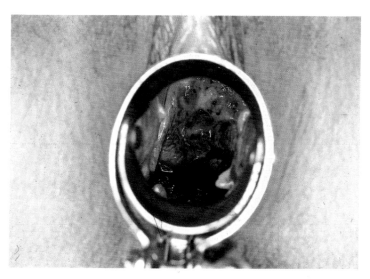

5.59

Figs 5.59–5.65 Exophytic Carcinoma. May
consist of small papillary excrescences (Figs 5.59,
5.60) or of cauliflower-like growths (Figs 5.61,
5.62). The surface vegetations are always friable
and bleed freely.

In the late stages the vagina may be filled with
a large cauliflower-like mass with variable degrees
of infiltration of the parametrium and/or the
vaginal walls. The tumour may occasionally be
relatively clean and uninfected (Fig. 5.63), but is
usually heavily infected, necrotic and may be
almost gangrenous (Figs 5.64, 5.65).

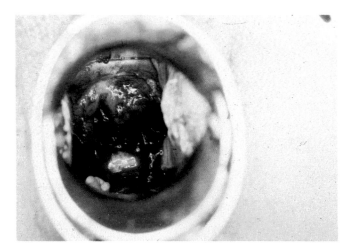

5.60

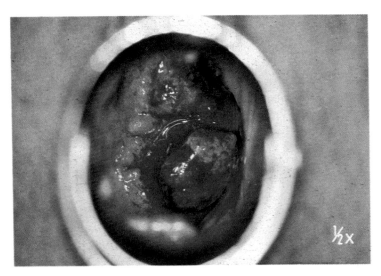

5.61

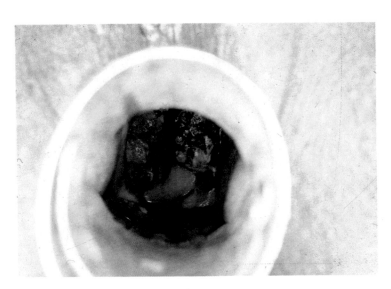

5.62

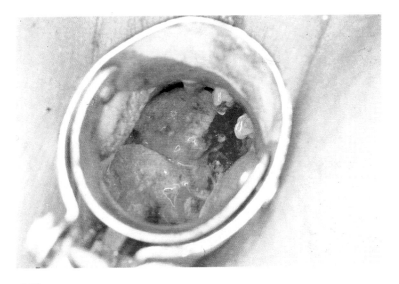

5.63

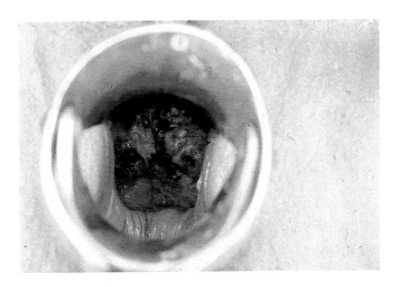

5.64

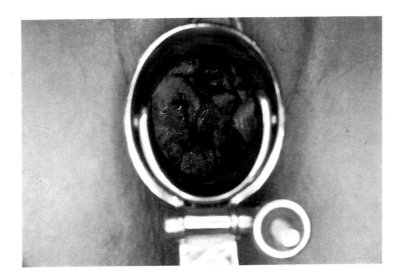

5.65

Colposcopy

Colposcopy is a most useful method for the detection of premalignant and early malignant lesions in the cervix and for choosing the best site for biopsy. Because there are a number of excellent colour atlases devoted to this technique[7,8] only a brief review of colposcopic appearances will be given. The diagrammatic representations are from the author's article on Colposcopy which was the first to be published on the subject in the British literature and are reproduced with the kind permission of the *Journal of Obstetrics and Gynaecology of the British Empire*.[9]

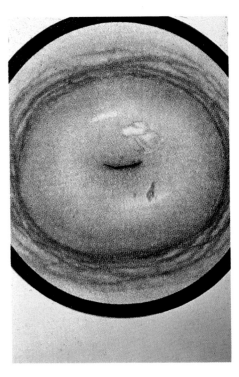

5.66

Fig. 5.66 Original Mucous Membrane. This is the typical squamous epithelium which is and has been originally present in this region. The squamous epithelium ends at the external os and is sharply limited from the columnar epithelium of the cervical canal. The mucous membrane appears pink and smooth all round and lacks the characteristic features which distinguish the other colposcopic pictures.

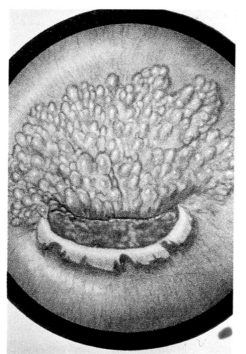

Fig. 5.67 Ectopia in Anterior Lip. Erosio Vera in Posterior Lip. Ectopia means the presence of columnar epithelium outside the external os. This has the appearance of grapes of variable size which swell on the application of 2% acetic acid. Erosio vera (true ulcer) is a raw area uncovered by epithelium. The latter is heaped up at the edge of the ulcer.

5.67

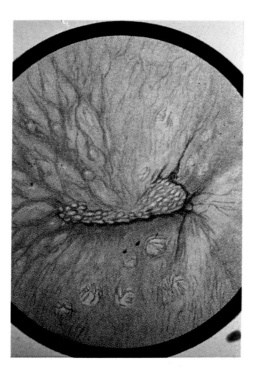

Fig. 5.68 Transformation Zone. This is an area of columnar epithelium (ectopia) being replaced by squamous epithelium. The growing squamous epithelium usually closes the orifices of glands present in the columnar epithelium with the formation of small Nabothian follicles covered by regularly branching blood vessels. The regular tree-like branching appearance of the blood vessels is an important feature of the normal transformation zone. Abnormalities of the blood vessels are an important feature of atypia and early malignancy.

5.68

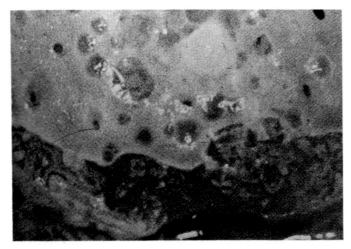

5.69

Fig. 5.69 Transformation Zone (colpophotograph). Note the squamous epithelium growing in tongue-like form over the ectopic area. The epithelium covering the glands has given way under the pressure of retained secretion resulting in the appearance of numerous small holes. These so called 'open glands' are another feature of the transformation zone.

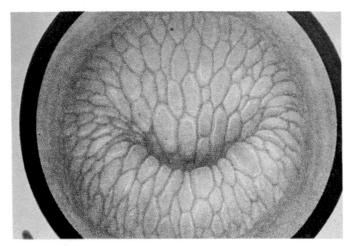

5.70

Fig. 5.70 Mosaic. This is a well-known appearance of atypical epithelium. In this case the mosaic surrounds the external os in circular fashion. The fields are regular in size and shape and are not raised above the surface; this usually signifies the presence of simple atypical epithelium. Marked irregularity and elevation of the mosaic areas indicate more pronounced degrees of atypia.

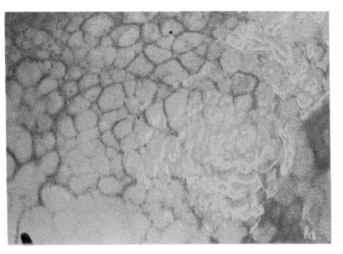

5.71

Fig. 5.71 Mosaic (colpophotograph).

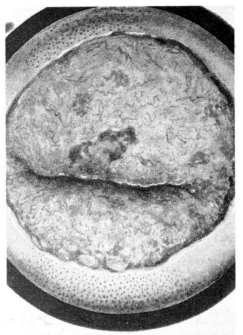

Fig. 5.72 Microcarcinoma. There are two areas to leukoplakic ground on the anterior and posterior lips at the edge of an extensive superficial ulcer surrounding the external os. Leukoplakic ground areas are smooth sharply demarcated iodine negative areas which show very fine red spots due to the presence of tiny capillary vessels at the tips of very fine papillae. These areas of atypical epithelium at the edge of a true ulcer, together with the marked irregularity of the blood vessels (comma-shaped and screw-like patterns), are strongly indicative of malignancy. Biopsy showed early invasive carcinoma.

5.72

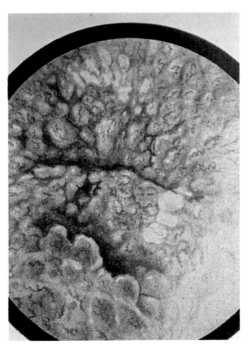

Fig. 5.73 Microcarcinoma. Irregular bossy elevations some of which appear glassy yellow in colour. Blood vessels irregular in size and shape. Small elevated leukoplakic patches are seen on the anterior lip. Biopsy showed early invasive carcinoma. The naked eye appearance of the cervix was not particularly suggestive.

5.73

6. Diseases of the Corpus Uteri and the Adnexa

Few abnormalities of the corpus uteri can be directly visualised. Two of these are the not uncommon fibroid polyp protruding through the cervix and the rare chronic inversion of the uterus.

A fibroid polyp is a submucous fibroid treated by the uterus as a foreign body and expelled through the dilated cervical canal. In the process it aquires a pedicle which can be traced up and found to arise from the uterine body, a point which differentiates it from cervical tumours and polypi. Colicky pains and bleeding are common symptoms of the fibroid polyp. Other differential diagnostic points are discussed in this chapter and in chapter 5.

A fibroid polyp sooner or later undergoes sloughing and necrosis causing a blood stained foul smelling discharge. An inexperienced examiner may mistake such a tumour, when of small size and present inside the cervix, for endocervical carcinoma. This serious and not uncommon pitfall is always avoidable. A fibroid polyp is never as friable as cervical carcinoma. More importantly, its origin, as mentioned above, can be traced to the inside of the uterine body. The most important diagnostic point is that endocervical carcinoma always infiltrates the adjacent tissues while in cases of fibroid polyp the finger can be passed freely around the tumour on all sides.

Still another diagnostic blunder is to mistake a fibroid polyp for chronic uterine inversion and *vice versa*. A fibroid polyp may very rarely be associated with and be actually the cause of chronic inversion by pulling on the uterine fundus. More commonly chronic inversion is a result of acute inversion complicating labour. Whatever the cause, chronic inversion can be recognized by the absence of the fundus uteri on bimanual examination. The diagnosis is confirmed by the careful passage of a uterine sound under aseptic conditions. In cases of chronic inversion of obstetric origin, the smooth surface and dark red colour of the inverted fundus are characteristic.

Laparoscopy, ultrasonography and radiography provide valuable means for 'indirect visualisation' of diseases of the corpus uteri and adnexa. These techniques are only very briefly discussed in this volume but references are given to excellent illustrated monographs describing the individual methods in great detail. It cannot be overemphasised that these useful techniques should be considered as an adjunct to and not as a substitute for careful history taking and meticulous examination. In lesions of the internal genital organs which cannot be directly seen, the physical signs elicited by palpation and sometimes by percussion are of the utmost importance. A description of these signs and their bearing on diagnosis is given in this chapter.

Fibroid polyp–Chronic inversion

Among the few diseases of the uterine body and the adnexa that may give rise to visible physical signs which can be photographed are uterine fibroid polypi and chronic inversion of the uterus.

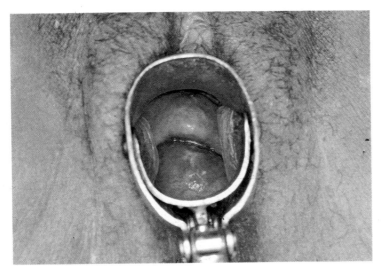

6.1

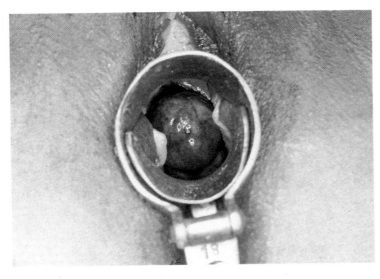

6.2

Figs 6.1–6.17 Fibroid Polyp. Uterine fibroid polypi may be expelled through the cervix, dilating the cervical canal as in labour or abortion. The tumour may be a solitary myoma or may appear to be formed of two or more amalgamated fibroids. They may by their sheer size, by acquiring a long pedicle or because of uterine descent actually appear at or outside the vulva. Infection and ulceration commonly complicate these tumours and the circulatory disturbances, caused by the tumour outgrowing its blood supply or by constriction of the pedicle, may result in sloughing and necrosis.

In Figs 6.1–6.3 the fibroid polyp is globular in shape and is formed of a solitary myoma. It protrudes into the upper part of the vagina and can only be visualized through a speculum. As previously mentioned, the globular shape of the tumour, its firm consistency and the rounded dilated appearance of the external os distinguish the fibroid polyp from the unusually large cervical mucous polyp.

In Figs 6.4–6.6 the fibroid polyp appears to be formed of more than one myoma and is somewhat irregular in shape. The bossy appearance of such tumours further helps to differentiate them from cervical polypi.

Fig. 6.7 Occasionally fibroid polypi may appear to be somewhat flattened and may much resembled in shape the large flattened fibroadenomatous mucous polyp of the cervix (see Figs 5.38, 5.39). In such cases microscopic examination may be the only way of determining the true nature of the tumour.

Figs. 6.8 & 6.9. Because of uterine descent a fibroid polyp, although not of very large size, may appear at the vulva. In both these cases the cervix is seen to be only a short distance above the vaginal introitus.

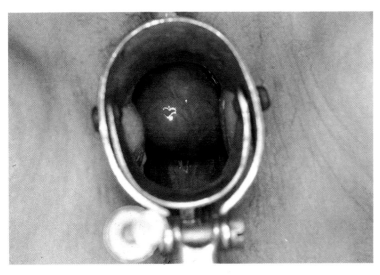

6.3

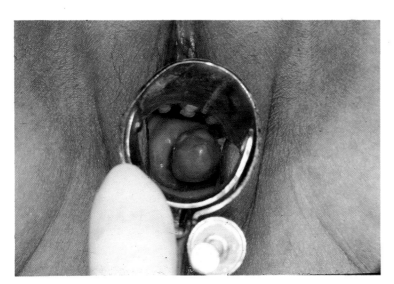

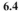

6.4

Fig. 6.10. A large fibroid polyp may reach down to the vulval level although the uterus is in normal position.

Fig. 6.11. Also by acquiring a long pedicle even a small or moderately sized fibroid polyp may appear at the vulva. In this case, because of torsion of the long pedicle, the tumour has become almost gangrenous.

Figs 6.12 & 6.13. Because of infection, sloughing and necrosis a fibroid polyp may superficially resemble the exophytic type of cervical carcinoma. The fibroid polyp, however, lacks the exuberant cauliflower-like formations of cervical carcinoma, shows much less friability, breakdown and ulceration and, most important of all, palpation reveals the high origin of the tumour and the absence of induration and infiltration of the walls of the cervix and vagina.

Figs 6.14 & 6.15. The hysterectomy specimen of the case shown in Fig. 6.13 shows the circumscribed nature of the tumour and the absence of any infiltration of the cervix.

Figs 6.16 & 6.17. Rarely large fibroid polypi, untreated for many years, acquire by metaplasia a covering of squamous epithelium similar to that of the vaginal walls which protects them from injury and infection.[10] These two illustrations show an example of this very unusual condition.

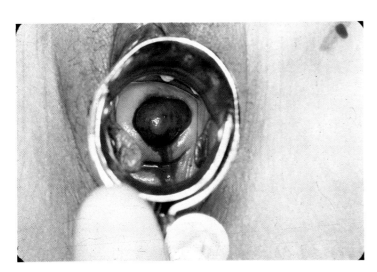

6.5

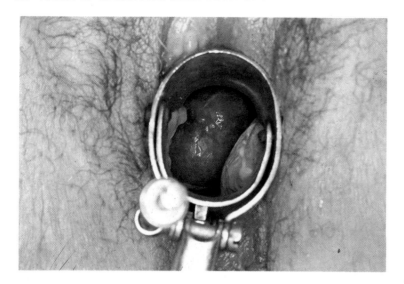

6.6

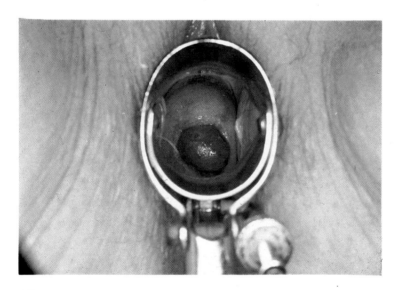

6.7

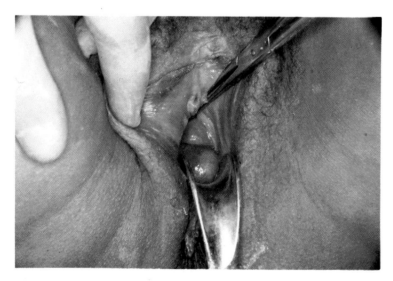

6.8

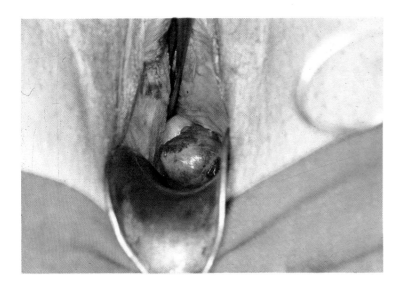

6.9

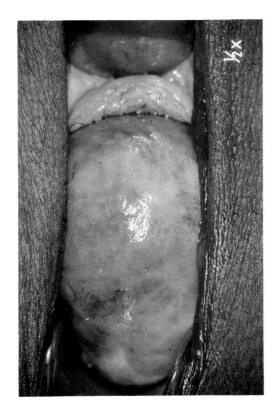

6.10

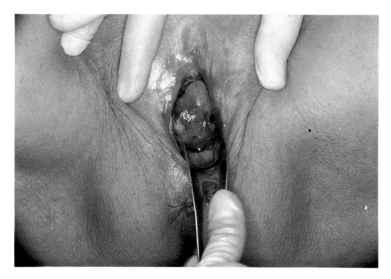

6.11

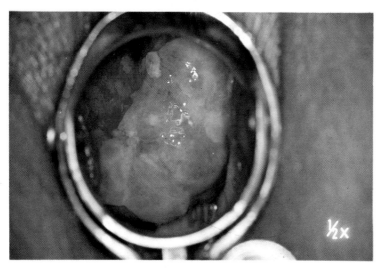

6.12

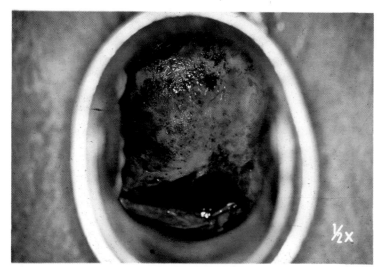

6.13

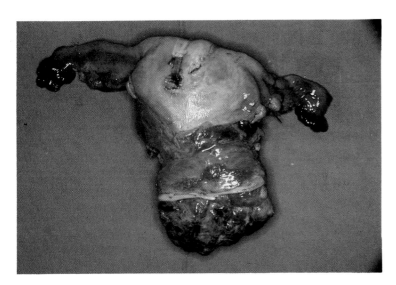

6.14

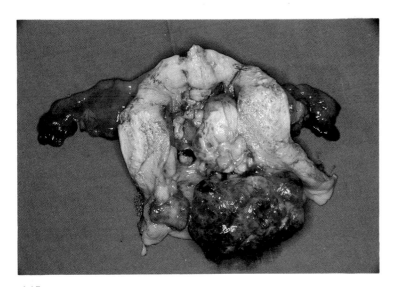

6.15

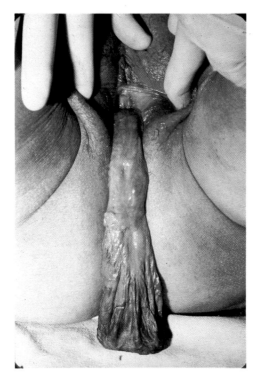

6.16

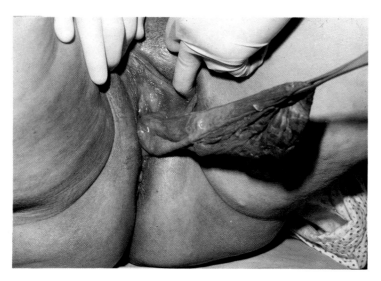

6.17

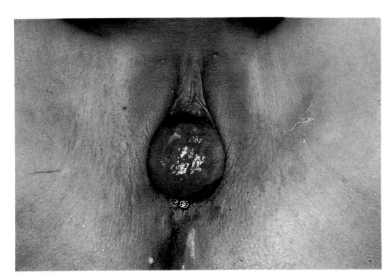

Fig. 6.18 Chronic Inversion of the Uterus. Here this rare complication resulted from untreated puerperal inversion. The patient complained of irregular uterine bleeding since her last labour one year before, and of a mass protruding from the vulva.

Note the smooth surface and the dark red colour of the inverted uterine fundus. The absence of the uterus on bimanual examination points to the correct diagnosis.

6.18

Some other diseases of the corpus and the adnexa

The conditions now discussed, as a rule, give rise to no visible physical signs except for abdominal enlargement caused by large swellings.

However, for the sake of completeness, a few illustrations of findings at laparotomy and of the specimens removed by operation are included to help explain some important diagnostic points.

The use of laparoscopy, ultrasonography and hysterosalpingography in the diagnosis of uterine and adnexal diseases will also be briefly discussed.

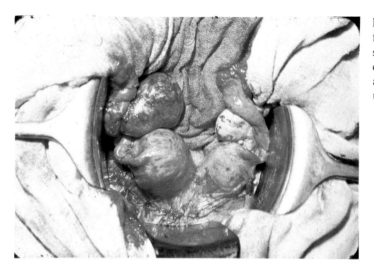

6.19

Fig. 6.19 Uterus Pseudodidelphys. In addition to finding two cervices and usually two vaginas, two separate uterine bodies can be felt on bimanual examination. As can be seen from the illustration, a tube and an ovary may be felt attached to each uterine body.

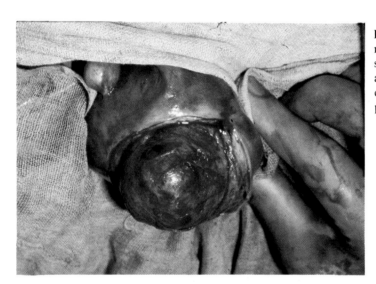

6.20

Fig. 6.20 Submucous Fibroid. This causes symmetrical enlargement of the uterus. It is often solitary. The uterus then feels smooth and regular and, especially if the fibroid is degenerated, the condition may be mistaken for normal or complicated pregnancy.

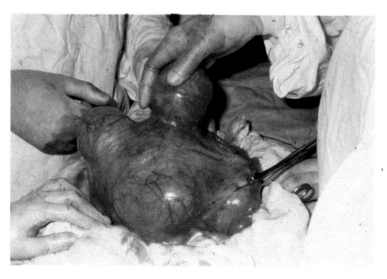

6.21

Figs 6.21–6.23 Multiple Uterine Fibroids. The bossy irregular surface of the swelling is an important diagnostic criterion. In spite of the multiplicity and large size of the tumours the uterine nature of the swelling can be recognized by 3 important physical signs: 1. The uterus cannot be felt separate from the tumour. 2. Movement of the abdominal mass causes movement of the cervix as felt by the fingers in the vagina.
3. Movement of the cervix with the vaginal fingers causes movement of the abdominal mass.

The commonest symptoms of fibroids are abnormal bleeding especially menorrhagia, pain, pressure symptoms, leucorrhoea and infertility.

Fig. 6.22 shows the surgical specimen removed from the case shown in Fig. 6.21.

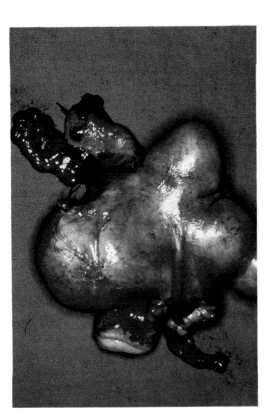

6.22

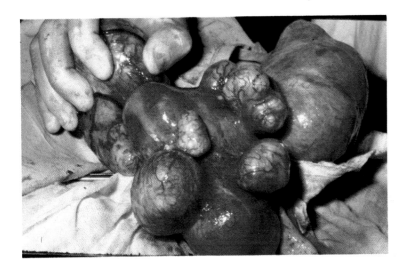

6.23

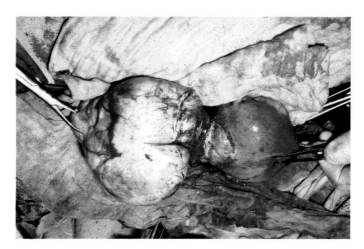

6.24

Fig. 6.24 Broad Ligament Fibroid. As can be seen in the illustration, broad ligament tumours can be felt separate from the uterus and they may displace it to the opposite side. The uterus itself may be normal in size. Patients with broad ligament myomata complain of pressure symptoms and pain rather than of abnormal bleeding.

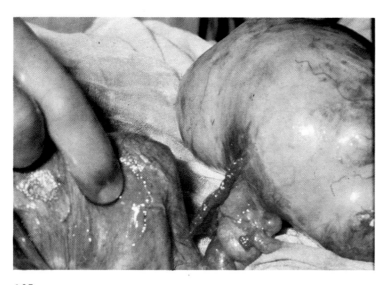

6.25

Fig. 6.25 Left Ovarian Tumour. The first point in the diagnosis of an ovarian tumour is to establish that the body of the uterus is felt separate from the tumour. Movement of the mass is not imparted to the cervix, and moving the cervix does not cause movement of the tumour.

The tumour usually has a smooth surface different from the bossy surface of a fibromyoma and may be cystic or solid.

Small and medium-sized cysts are usually felt lateral to or behind the uterus with their lower pole in the pouch of Douglas, but a dermoid cyst or a solid tumour may, by its weight, come to lie anteriorly.

Ovarian tumours may be symptomless or the patient may complain of pain, pressure symptoms and/or abdominal swelling. Menstrual disorders are not common except in functioning and malignant tumours.

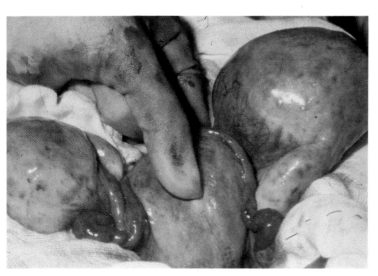

6.26

Fig. 6.26 Bilateral Overian Dermoid Cysts. When the cysts are small, as in the case shown, it is possible to distinguish two quite separate tumours on two distinctly separate pedicles. But large tumours with irregular configuration may show segmentations which may give rise to the false assumption that a bilateral tumour is present.

Bilateral tumours are often, but by no means always, malignant. In the case shown they appear freely mobile and none of the signs of malignancy (see below) are present. They proved to be innocent dermoid cysts.

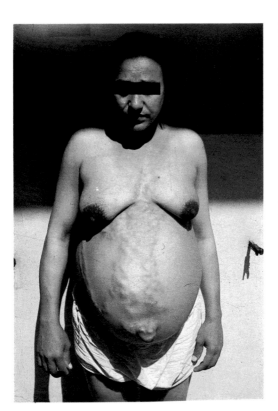

6.27

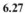

Figs 6.27 & 6.28 Malignant Ovarian Tumour, Ascites. Varicose Veins. In cases of ovarian tumour ascites is almost always an indication of malignancy, but ascites and even hydrothorax may occasionally be associated with benign tumours such as ovarian fibroma (Meigs Syndrome).

In the case shown there was also marked enlargement and varicosity of the veins in the anterior abdominal wall and in the right leg and thigh. Varicose veins and/or oedema of the lower limb especially when unilateral in a case of ovarian tumour are strongly suggestive of malignancy.

Other signs of possible malignancy in ovarian tumour cases are rapid growth, cachexia and solidity, fixity and bilaterality of the tumour. The presence of metastatic nodules in the parietal peritoneum, liver or Douglas pouch is sure evidence of malignancy.

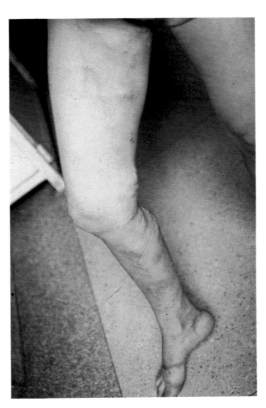

6.28

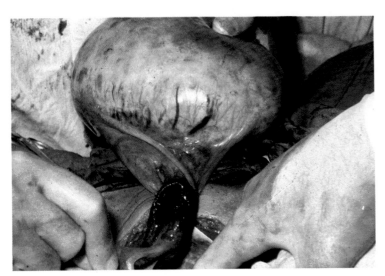

6.29

Figs 6.29 & 6.30 Torsion of Ovarian Cyst. The physical signs of ovarian cyst are the same as already described. In addition, there is marked tenderness of the tumour and rigidity of the lower abdomen.

The symptoms are severe pain of rapid onset and may be shock, vomiting and later pyrexia.

Note the gangrenous pedicle and the haemorrhage inside the tumour. Fig. 6.30 shows the cyst after removal.

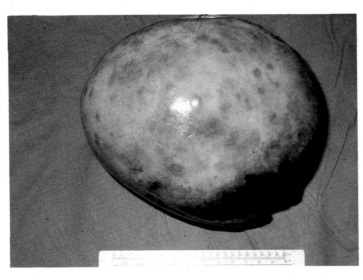

6.30

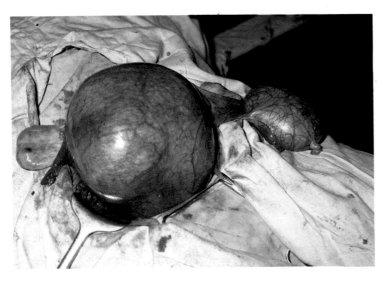

6.31

Figs 6.31 & 6.32 Small Parovarian Cyst. Uterine Fibroids. The clinician should be careful not to miss the presence of more than one tumour in the same patient.

In the case shown there were multiple uterine fibroids, the diagnosis of which presented no difficulty. Also present was a small right parovarian cyst. The latter is recognized, as can be seen in the illustration, by the ovary being felt separate from the cyst, which cannot therefore be ovarian, and by the Fallopian tube being stretched on its top. These cysts cause few symptoms except if they become twisted or infected.

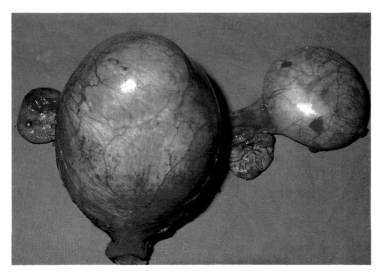

6.32

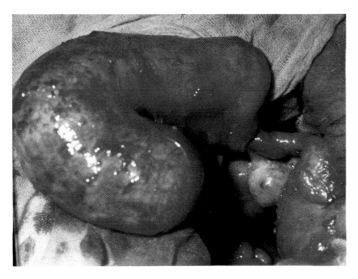

6.33

Figs 6.33 & 6.34 Hydrosalpinx. A large hydrosalpinx is felt bimanually as a swelling separate from both uterus and ovary, usually bilateral, tender, somewhat fixed and has the typical retort shape seen in the illustrations.

A pyosalpinx shows similar signs but the tenderness and fixity are much more marked and its much thicker walls give the impression of a firm swelling.

If the ovary shares in the inflammatory process the condition is known as tuboovarian cyst or tuboovarian abscess. The retort shape of the hydrosalpinx or pyosalpinx is then lost and the mass becomes more or less globular or spherical.

The symptoms and signs of active pelvic infection are much more marked in pyosalpinx than in hydrosalpinx. These include foul vaginal discharge, recurrent attacks of pain and pyrexia, leucocytosis and high sedimentation rate.

A small hydrosalpinx may not be clinically palpable and its only symptom may be infertility. The diagnosis can then be made by lapaparoscopy and/or hysterosalpingography (see pp. 167, 173). These methods are also very helpful in the diagnosis of cases of genital tuberculosis.

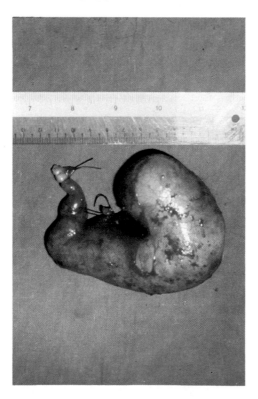

6.34

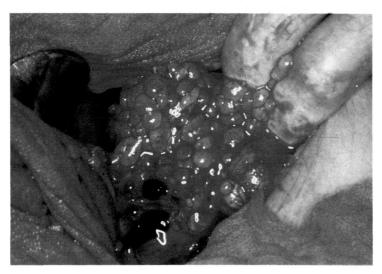

Figs 6.35 & 6.36 Hydatidiform Mole. This obstetric complication is included because it is not infrequently mistaken for a large degenerated submucous myoma. In both conditions there is a softish symmetrical uterine swelling and bleeding may be a prominent symptom.

In hydatidiform mole there may be history of amenorrhoea and other pregnancy symptoms, vomiting may be excessive and the blood pressure may be high. The abdominal swelling has a characteristic doughy feeling on palpation and one or both ovaries may be grossly cystic. Occasionally the patient or the doctor may notice the passage per vaginam of the characteristic vesicles seen in the illustrations. Hormonal tests and/or ultrasonography may be carried out to establish the diagnosis.

6.35

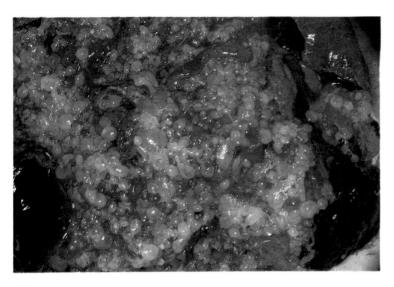

6.36

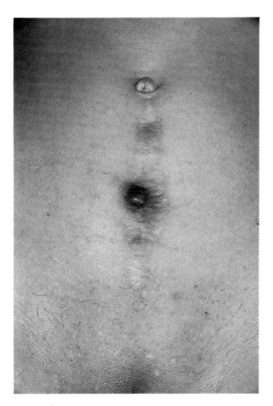

6.37

Figs 6.37 & 6.38 Endometriosis of Laparotomy Scar. A plum coloured swelling in the scar line which usually becomes large, more painful and tender at the time of menstruation due to congestion, oedema and possibly bleeding in the ectopic endometrial tissue.

In the case shown in Fig. 6.37 the condition occurred after classical Caesarean section performed by a general surgeon and in the case in Fig. 6.38 after abdominal myomectomy.

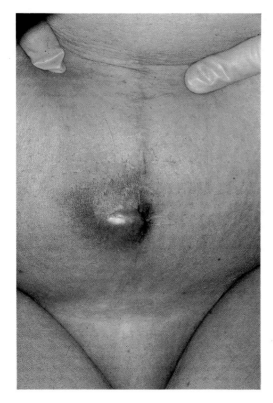

6.38

Laparoscopy

There are very good illustrated works devoted to laparoscopy,[11,12] ultrasonography,[13,14] and hysterosalpingography.[15,16] Only a brief presentation of these techniques will therefore be included to show some of their possible applications in gynaecological diagnosis.

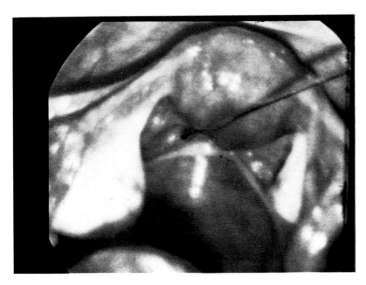

6.39

Fig. 6.39 Normal Laparoscopic Appearances.

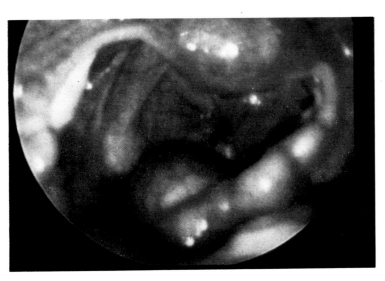

6.40

Fig. 6.40 Bilateral Small Hydrosalpinx. Note the retort shape and posterior position of the distended tube. The condition is more marked on the right side.

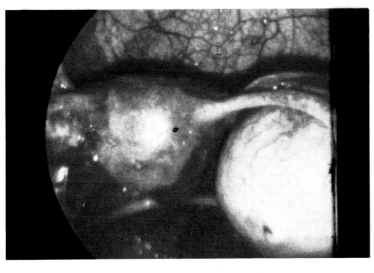

6.41

Fig. 6.41 Small Cystoma Simplex of the Right Ovary.

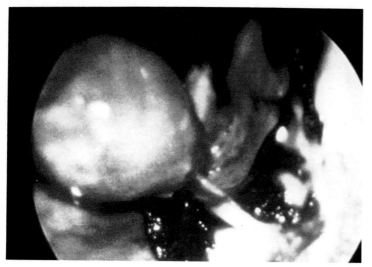

Fig. 6.42 Right Tubal Pregnancy. Early Rupture. Note the blood oozing from the site of rupture.

The symptoms of tubal pregnancy are pain and bleeding usually after a period of amenorrhoea. There is exquisite tenderness over the affected tube which may be palpably swollen and on palpation of the posterior fornix which may be distended with a pelvic haematocele. The diagnosis of ectopic pregnancy represents one of the most useful applications of laparoscopy.

6.42

Ultrasonography

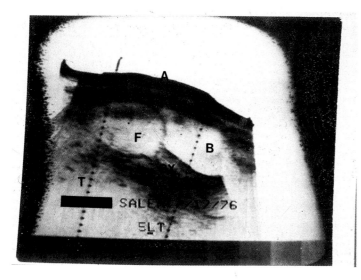

Fig. 6.43 Submucous Myoma. Longitudinal scan showing almost uniform enlargement of the uterine fundus. This echographic pattern points to the possible presence of a submucous myoma. B = bladder; F = fibroid uterus; CX = cervix uteri; A = anterior abdominal wall; T = tracer centimetre marker (longitudinal grey scale scan).

6.43

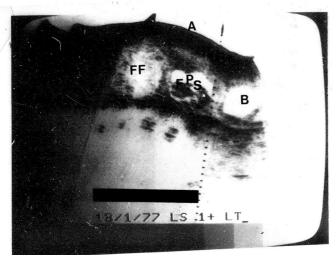

Fig. 6.44 Early Pregnancy. Fundal Myoma.
Longitudinal scan showing an early intrauterine pregnancy sac. Perched on the sac is a relatively anechoic circular area of a fundal myoma. A = anterior abdominal wall; B = bladder; P = placenta; S = amniotic sac; F = fetal parts; FF = fundal fibroid (longitudinal grey scale scan).

6.44

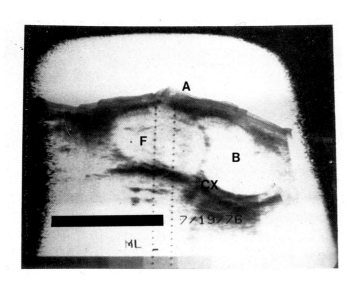

Fig. 6.45 Uterine Fibroid. Hyaline Degeneration.
Longitudinal scan showing almost uniform enlargement of the uterine fundus. Good sound penetration is demonstrated giving echographic evidence of a degenerative process. Note the continuity of the mass with the cervix and vagina indicating its uterine origin. A = anterior abdominal wall; B = bladder; F = fibroid uterus; CX = cervix uteri (longitudinal grey scale scan).

6.45

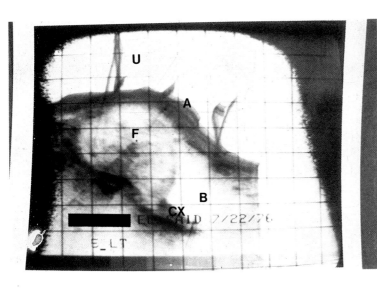

Fig. 6.46 Multiple Uterine Fibroids. Longitudinal scan revealing uterine enlargement. Note the irregular outline of the uterus, an echographic pattern corresponding to the clinical feeling of bossy uterus on palpation. This is the typical sonographic picture of multiple uterine fibroids. A = anterior abdominal wall; B = bladder; F = bossy leiomyomators uterous; U = umbilical region (longitudinal grey scale scan).

6.46

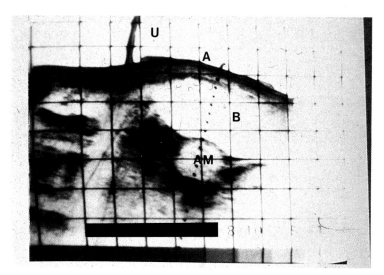

6.47

Fig. 6.47 Chocolate Cyst of Ovary. Longitudinal lateral pelvic scan revealing an adnexal mass that is relatively echo-free. A grid system for echographic measurement is co-projected. The mass proved to be a chocolate cyst of the ovary. A = anterior abdominal wall; U = umbilicus; B = bladder; AM = adnexal mass (endometriosis of the ovary) (longitudinal scan).

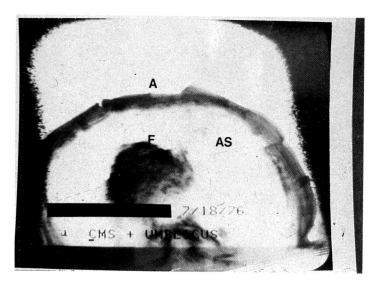

6.48

Fig. 6.48 Fibroma of the Ovary. Longitudinal abdominal scan showing large anechoic limitless areas denoting the presence of free ascitic fluid. In the middle of the fluid there is an echogenic blackish area of a solid tumour. This proved to be a case of ovarian fibroma with ascites (Meigs syndrome). A = anterior abdominal wall; AS = ascitic fluid; F = fibroma of the ovary (transverse grey scale scan).

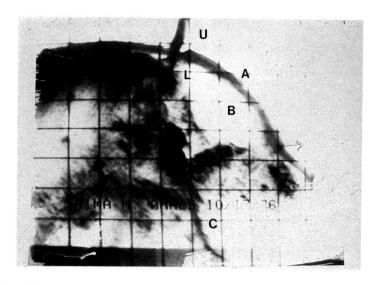

6.49

Fig. 6.49 Carcinoma of the Ovary. Bizarre echographic pattern of advanced ovarian malignancy revealed in longitudinal scan. A mixture of pocketed ascitic fluid, bowel black echoes and dome of the ovarian tumour is displayed. A = anterior abdominal wall; U = umbilicus; AS = ascitic fluid; L = loops of bowel amalgamated with omentum; B = bladder; C = ovarian mass (carcinoma) (longitudinal grey scale scan).

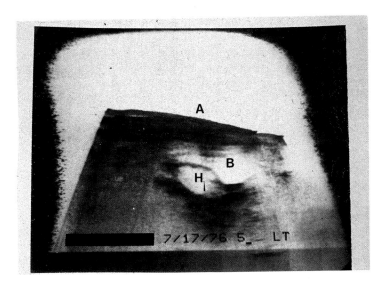

Fig. 6.50 Hydrosalpinx. Lateral longitudinal scan showing an oblong thin walled anechoic adnexal mass. This proved, as expected, to be a hydrosalpinx. A = anterior abdominal wall; B = bladder; H = hydrosalpinx (longitudinal grey scale scan).

6.50

Hysterosalpingography

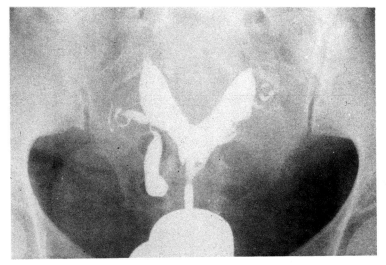

6.51

Figs 6.51–6.53 Diagnosis of Congenital Anomalies of the Uterus.
Fig. 6.51 Uterus Septus.
Fig. 6.52 Uterus Bicornis Unicollis.
Fig. 6.53 Uterus Pseudodidelphys.

The latter condition is differentiated from the former by the lower level and much wider angle of separation, and by the convex appearance of the medial border of the cornu in uterus bicornis (Fig. 6.52) as compared with the straight medial border in uterus septus (Fig. 6.51).

Fig. 6.53 Uterus Pseudodidelphys. Two cervices and two uterine bodies. See Fig. 6.19 for the appearance at operation.

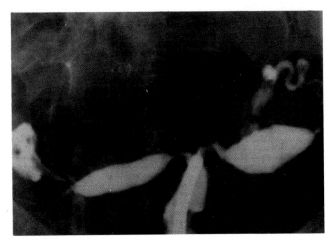

6.52

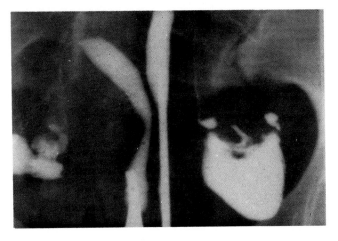

6.53

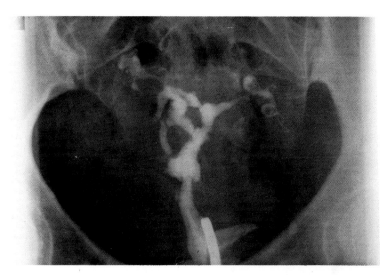

6.54

Figs 6.54–6.56 Investigation of Infertility.

Fig. 6.54 Intrauterine Synechia. These may be associated with hypomenorrhoea and infertility. Note the irregular filling defects.

Fig. 6.55 Bilateral Hydrosalpinx. Tubal block is a common cause of infertility. Note the dilatation of the ampullary part of the tube on both sides. Such a small hydrosalpinx cannot be recognized by clinical palpation.

Fig. 6.56 Bilateral Interstitial Tubal Block. Intravasation. Bilateral block at the uterine end of the tube on both sides. Note maked intravasation.

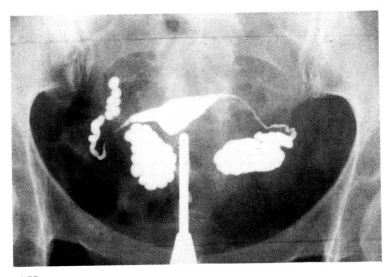

6.55

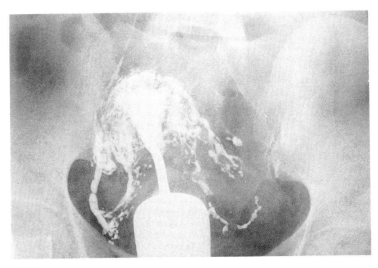

6.56

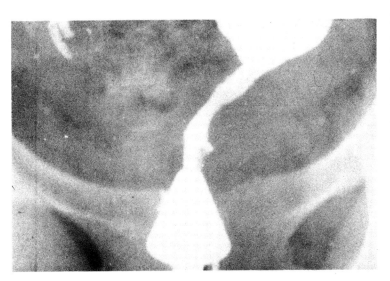

6.57

Fig. 6.57 Investigation of Mid-Trimester Abortion. In such cases isthmography should be carried out in the luteal phase of the cycle when the isthmus is normally norrow and its sphincters are tightly closed.[17]

In the case shown the isthmus is abnormally wide with no appearent constriction at its upper or lower borders, an appearance diagnostic of incompetent isthmus.

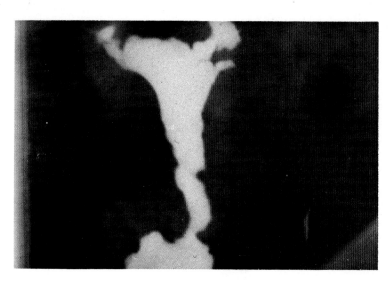

6.58

Figs 6.58 & 6.59 Investigation of Uterine Bleeding.

Fig. 6.58 Two small uterine polypi are seen, one at either cornu. These cannot of course be diagnosed by uterine palpation and may even be missed at curettage.

Fig. 6.59 Note the characteristic crescentic appearance of the uterine cavity in cases of submucous myoma.

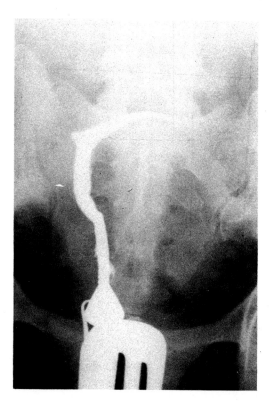

6.59

References

1. International Society for the Study of Vulval Disease 1976 New nomenclature for vulval disease Obstetrics and Gynecology 47:122
2. Way S 1982 Malignant Disease of the Vulva Edinburgh-London: Churchill Livingstone
3. Gardner H L and Kaufman R H 1981 Benign Diseases of the Vulva and Vagina Boston Mass: Hall Medical Publishers
4. Youssef A F 1960 editor Gynecological Urology Springfield Illinois: Charles C Thomas
5. Youssef A F and Shukry M I 1969 Abortion in Duplications of the Uterus The Role of Associated Isthmic Incompetence Ain Shams Medical Journal 20:445
6. Navratil E 1964 In Dysplasia Carcinoma in Situ and Microinvasive Carcinoma of the Cervix edited by Gray L A Springfield Illinois: Charles C Thomas
7. Cramer H 1956 Die Kolposkopie in der Praxis Stuttgart: Thieme
8. Dexeus S Garrera J M and Coupez F 1977 Colposcopy Philadelphia: Saunders
9. Youssef A F 1957 Colposcopy The results of its routine employment in 1000 gynaecological patients Journal of Obstetrics and Gynaecology of the British Empire 64:801
10. MacLeod D H and Read C D 1955 Gynaecology fifth edition London: Churchill
11. Semm K 1976 Pelviskopie und Hysteroskopie Stuttgart: Schattaver
12. Steptoe P C 1967 Laparoscopy in Gynaecology Edinburgh: Livingstone
13. Athey P A Hadlock F P 1981 Ultrasound in obstetrics and gynecology St Louis: Mosby
14. Schlensker K H 1975 Atlas of Ultrasonic Diagnosis in Obstetrics and Gynecology Stuttgart: Thieme
15. Dalsace J and Garcia-Galderon J 1959 Gynecologic Radiography New York: Hoeber-Harper
16. Siegler A M 1967 Hysterosalpingography New York: Harper and Row
17. Youssef A F 1958 The Uterine Isthmus and its Sphincter Mechanism A Radiographic Study American Journal of Obstetrics and Gynecology 75:1305 1320

Index

Abortion, mid-trimester,
  hysterosalpingography, 173
Adenomatous type of mucous polyp, 132
Adrenal hyperplasia, congenital, 2
Allergic dermatitis, right labium majus, 16
Allergic ulcers, labia, 26, 27
Amenorrhoea, false, vagina, 60
Androgen ingestion and intersexuality, 2
Aplasia, vagina, 62–63
Ascites and malignant ovarian tumour, 161
Atresia, vagina, 68

Bartholin cyst, 30–34
Behçet's syndrome, 22, 23
Benign tumours
  cervix, 135, 136
  corpus, 158–160, 162–163
  ovary, 160
  vagina, 78–80
  vulva, 37–42
Bilharzial
  carcinoma, vaginal, 81
  papillomata, multiple large, labia majus,
    20–21
  vagina, 71, 72
Bilharziasis, cervix, 124
Bleeding uterine, hysterosalpingography,
  174
Bowen's disease, 43

Carcinoma
  cervix uteri, 138–143
  ovarian, ultrasonography, 170
  urethral, 57, 58
  vaginal, 80–81
    Bilharzial, 81
  vulva 44–51
  vulvo-urethral, 58
Cervix uteri, diseases, 120–147
  benign tumours, 135, 136
    suspicious, 136, 137
  bilharziasis, 124
  carcinoma, 138–143
    advanced, 139–141
    exophytic, 141–143
    stage I, 138–139
    ulcerative, 140, 141
  cervicovaginal fistula, anterior, 122
    posterior, 121
  colposcopy, 144–147
    ectopia in anterior lip, 145
    erosio vera in posterior lip, 145
    microcarcinoma, 147

mosaic, 146
    original mucous membrane, 144
    transformation zone, 145, 146
  congenital, 120
    duplication, 120
    elongation, 121
  double, 65
  erosion, 120, 125–129
    follicular (cystic), 127
    healing, 128
    papillary, 126–127
    in a pill user, 128
    in pregnancy, 127
    simple flat, 125–126
    starting polyp formation, 129
  examination, 120
  in infertility, 120
  polyp, 120, 130–134
    mucous, 130—134
    with prolapse, 95
  prolapse, 88–102
    elongation and hypertrophy, 99
      recurrent, 101
    erosion, 95
    pigmentation, 94
    ulceration, 96, 97
  tear, bilateral, 122
    ectropion, 123
      with uterine prolapse, 123
  tumours, benign, 135
  ulcer, 124
    and vagina, 124
Choriocarcinoma, metastatic
  vagina, 82
  vulval, 52
Circumcision, female, adhesions, 6–7
  epidermoid cyst after, 27–30
Clitoris, hypertrophy, 2–4
Colposcopy, 144–147
Condylomata acuminata, 19
Condylomata lata, 20
Congenital adrenal hyperplasia, 2
Congenital anomalies
  cervix, 120
  corpus, 158, 171, 172
  vagina, 60–67
  vulva, 2–4
Contraceptive pill, oral, and cervical
  erosion, 128
Corpus uteri and adnexa, diseases, 149–174
  chronic inversion, 149, 157
  endometriosis of laparotomy scar, 165,
    166

fibroid polyp, 149–156
  diagnosis, 149
fibroids, 158–160
hydatiform mole, 164, 165
hydrosalpinx, 163, 164
hysterosalpingography, 171–174
laparoscopy, 149, 157, 166–168
ovarian cysts, 160, 162–163
ovarian tumour, 161
  left, 160
    malignant, with ascites and varicose
      veins, 161
  uterus pseudodidelphys, 65, 158, 171, 172
  radiography, 149, 157
  ultrasonography, 149, 157, 168–170
Cryptomenorrhoea, 60
Cystic type of mucous polyp, 132
Cystocele, 9
  anterior vaginal wall, 86, 88
  in nullipara, 92
Cystorectocele, 91, 100
Cysts
  ovarian, chocolate, 170
    dermoid, bilateral, 160
    small parovarian and uterine fibroids,
      162, 163
    torsion, 162
  urethral, 56
  vagina, 59, 72–77
    Gaertner, 72–75
    posterior wall, 76–77
  vulva, 27–36
    Bartholin, 30–34
    epidermoid, 27–30
    hymenal, 34, 35
    sebaceous, 35–36

Dermatitis, allergic, right labium majus, 16
Dermoid cysts, bilateral ovarian, 160
Diffuse capillary haemangioma, cervix, 135
Dystrophy, vulval, 9

Ectopic pregnancy, 168
Ectopia vesica, 117
Endometriosis of laparotomy scar, 165, 166
Enterocele, 94
Epidermoid cysts, labia, 27–30
Epithelioma, vulva
  endophytic or ulcerative, 44–46
    recurrent, 50
  exophytic or fungoid, 47–48
    recurrent, 51

Epithelioma, vulva *(cont'd)*
  involving lymph nodes, 49
    recurrent, 50, 51

Fibroadenomatous type of mucous polyp,
  133
Fibroid polyp, 149–156
Fibroids, uterine
  with parovarian cyst, 162, 163
  submucous, 158
    broad ligament, 160
    multiple, 158–159
  ultrasonography, 169
    hyaline degeneration, 169
    multiple, 169
Fibroma
  cervical, 135, 136
  vaginal, 79
    vesicovaginal septum, 80
  vulval, 40, 41
Fibrosarcoma, vaginal, 82
Fistulas
  genitourinary, 103, 110–117
    urethro vaginal, 110–112
    vesicovaginal, 112–117
      vulvitis, 115
  posterior cervicovaginal, 121
  rectovaginal, 103, 108–109, 117
    with large vesicovaginal fistula, 117
    vestibular anus, 109
Follicular (cystic) erosion, 127
Foreign body causing vaginal ulcer, 70

Gaertner cysts, vagina, 72–75
Genital prolapse, 85–102
  see also Prolapse, genital
Genitourinary fistulas, 103, 110–117
  urethro vaginal, 110–112
  vesicovaginal, 112–117
    vulvitis, 115
Granulation tissue, septic, at vaginal vault,
  70
Granuloma inguinale, 23

Haemangioma, diffuse capillary, cervix, 135
Haematocolpos, vagina, 60–62
Haematoma, vaginal, 69
Haematometra, 60
Hernia, bilateral inguinal, 9
Herpes simplex, labia, 24, 25
Hidradenoma, labia, 38
Hydatidiform moles, 164, 165
Hydrosalpinx, 163, 164
  hysterosalpingography, 172
  laparoscopy, 167
Hymenal cysts, 34, 35
Hyperplastic dystrophy, 9
Hypertrophy, clitoris, 2–4
Hysterectomy, total, abdominal, vault
  prolapse after, 93
Hysterosalpingography, 171–174
  infertility investigation, 172, 173
  mid-trimester abortion, investigation, 173
  uterine bleeding, investigation, 174
  uterus, congenital anomalies, 171–172

Infertility, hysterosalpingography, 172, 173
Inflammation, vaginal, 68–71
  vulval, 68–71
Intersexuality, 2–4
Intertrigo, 13
Intrauterine synechia,
  hysterosalpingography, 172

Intravasation, uterine,
  hysterosalpingography, 172
Isthmus, incompetence of, 173

Labia
  adhesions, 4–5
    following burn, 7
    following circumcision, 6
    post-traumatic, 5
  cysts, 27–36
  fusion, 1
  inflammation, 9–26
  minora, elongation, 4
  skin affections, 9–26
  tumours, benign solid, 37–42
    malignant, 43–53
  ulcers, 26
Labiascrotal fusion, 3–4
Laparoscopy, 149, 157, 166–168
  bilateral small hydrosalpinx, 167
  normal appearances, 167
  right tubal pregnancy, 168
  small cystoma simplex, ovary, 167
Laparotomy scar, endometriosis, 165, 166
Leukoderma, 13–16
Leukoplakia, 9–12
  definition, 9
Lichen planus, 12
Lichen sclerosus, 12
Lipoma, labia, 39–40
Lymphangioma circumscriptum, labia, 42

Melanoma, malignant
  vaginal, 83
  vulval, 53
Menouria (Youssef's syndrome), 103
Microcarcinoma, cervix uteri, 147
Monilia vaginitis, 70
Monilia vulvitis, 17–18
Mucous cervical polyp, 130–134
  adenomatous type, 132
  cystic type, 132
  fibroadenomatous type, 133
  large, 133, 134
  multiple, 131
  necrotic, 134
Myoma, submucous, ultrasonography, 168
  fundal, early pregnancy, 169
Myoma, uterine *see* Fibroids

Neurofibromatosis, multiple, labia, 41, 42

Oedema, vulval, 8
Ovary
  small cystoma simplex, right, 167
  tumour, left, 160
    bilateral dermoid cysts, 160
  ultrasonography, fibroma, 170
    carcinoma, 170

Papillary cervical erosion, 126–127
Papillomata
  Bilharzial, multiple large, 20–21, 71, 72
  true, 37–38, 79
Perineal tears, 103–108
  complete, 104–108
  incomplete, 103, 104
Pigmentation
  in prolapse, 94
  vagina, 69
Piles, 9

Polyp
  cervical, with prolapse, 95
    formation, starting from cervical
      erosion, 129
    mucous, 130–134
      see also Mucous cervical polyp
  fibroid, 149–156
  vaginal, 78
Pouch of Douglas, hernia, 94
Pre-eclampsia causing vulval oedema, 8
Pregnancy
  cervical erosion in, 127
  early, fundal myoma, ultrasonography, 169
  tubal, right, laparoscopy, 168
Procidentia, 89–91
Prolapse, genital, 85–102
  cervix, erosion, 95
    polyp, 95
    see also Cervix uteri, prolapse
  cystocele, 86, 88
  elongation and hypertrophy, cervix, 99
    recurrent, 100
  enterocele, 94
  examination, 85
  nulliparous, 91, 92
  pigmentation in, 94
  posterior vaginal wall, 86, 88
  rectocele, 86
  rectum, 100
  recurrent, 101–102
  ulceration, 96, 97
    cervix, 96, 97
  uterine with ectropion, 123
  uterus, 87–91, 100
    recurrent, 101
  vault, after hysterectomy, 93
    recurrent, 102
Pseudodidelphys, uterus, 65, 158
  hysterosalpingography, 171, 172
Pseudohermaphroditism, female, 3

Rectocele, 86
Rectovaginal fistulas, 103, 108–109, 117
  vestibular anus, 109

Sebaceous cyst, labia, 35–36
Synechia, intrauterine,
  hysterosalpingography, 172
Synechia vulvae, 4, 5
Syphilis, primary, labium majus, 23

Tears
  cervical, bilateral, 122
    ectropion, 123
      with uterine prolapse, 123
    right, 122
  perineal, 103–108
Tubal block, interstitial, bilateral,
  hysterosalpingography, 172
Tubal pregnancy, right, laparoscopy, 168

Ulcers
  allergic, labia, 26
  cervix, 124
  infected traumatic, labia, 26
  non-specific inflammatory, labia, 25
  and prolapse, vagina, 95
    cervix, 96, 97
    vulva, 98
  vaginal, 68–71, 95
    caused by foreign body, 70
    extensive, 69

Ultrasonography, 149, 157, 168–170
    fibroids, 169
    fundal myoma in early pregnancy, 169
    ovary, chocolate cyst, 170
        carcinoma, 170
        fibroma, 170
    submucous myoma, 168
Urethral diseases, 53–58
    carcinoma, 57, 58
    caruncle, 53–55
    cyst, 56
    prolapse, 56, 57
Urethrovaginal fistula, 110–112
Uterus
    bicornis bicollis, 120
        unicollis, hysterosalpingography, 171,
            172
    bleeding, hysterosalpingography, 174
    chronic inversion, 149, 157
    double (pseudodidelphys), 65, 158, 171,
        172
    hysterosalpingography, 171–172
        bicornis unicollis, 171, 172
        pseudodidelphys, 171, 172
        septus, 171, 172
    prolapse, first degree, 87–88
        second degree, 88–89
        in nullipara, 92
        third degree, 89–91, 100
            differentiation from second, 89–91
        see also Cervix uteri; Prolapse
    septus, hysterosalpingography, 171, 172
    see also Cervix uteri; Corpus uteri

Vagina, diseases, 59–83
    aplasia, 62–63

atresia, 68
carcinoma, 59, 80–82
congenital, 59, 60–67
cysts, 59, 72–77
double, 64, 65
inflammation, 59, 67–72
longitudinal septum, partial, 64
    complete, 64–67
posterior wall prolapse, 86, 88
prolapse, pigmentation, 94
    ulceration, 95, 97
septic granulation tissue at vault, 70
tumours, 59
    benign, 78–80
    malignant, 80–83
ulcers, 68–71
    and of cervix, 124
Vaginitis, monilia, 70
    senile, 71
Varicose veins and malignant ovarian
    tumour, 161
Varicosities, vulval, 7–8
Vesicovaginal
    fistula, 112–117
        vulvitis, 115
    septum, fibroma, 80
Vitiligo see Leukoderma
Von Recklinghausen's disease, labia, 41, 42
Vulva, diseases of, 1–58
    allergic dermatitis, 16
    bilharziasis, 20, 21
    condylomata, 19, 20
    congenital anomalies, 2–4
    cysts
        Bartholin, 30–34
        epidermoid, 27–30

hymenal, 34, 35
    sebaceous, 35, 36
dystrophy, 9–11
examination, 1
intertrigo, 13
labial adhesions, 4–7
leukoderma, 13–16
leukoplakia, 9–11
lichen, 12
monilia, 17, 18
nonspecific inflammation, 16, 17
oedema, 8
tumours, benign
    fibroma, 40, 41
    hidradenoma, 38
    lipoma, 39, 40
    lymphangioma, 42, 43
    neurofibroma, 41, 42
    papilloma, 37, 38
tumours, malignant
    Bowen's disease, 43
    choriocarcinoma, 52
    epithelioma
        endophytic, 44–46
        exophytic, 47, 48
        lymph node metastases, 49
        recurrent, 50, 51
    melanoma, 53
    ulcers, 22–27
    varicosities, 7, 8
Vulvitis
    acute non-specific, 16, 17
    monilia, 17–18
Vulvourethral carcinoma, 58

Youssef's syndrome, 103